Intermittent Fasting

as a Lifestyle

Mia Walker

Guide for you that will help you quickly and easily build up a Healthy and Beautiful Body

Your Free Gift

I would like to show my appreciation that you support my work so I've put together a free gift for you that can be found at the link

http://ehpcom.com/

7 Day-Meal

I know you will love this gift.

Thanks!

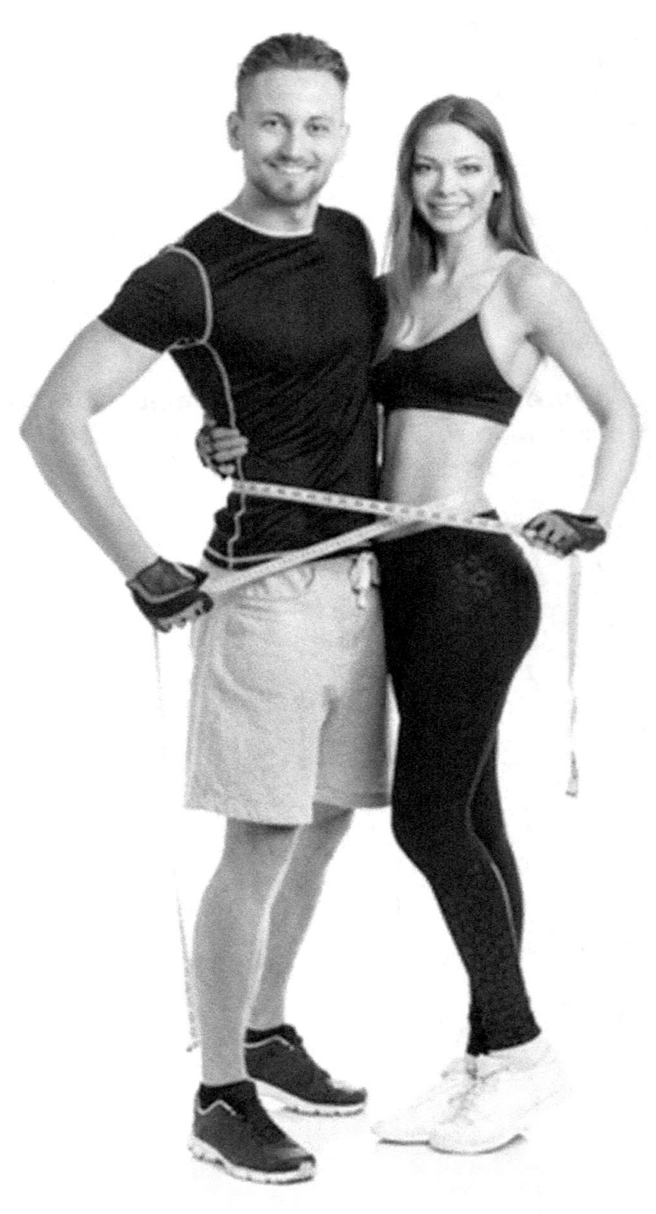

Contents

Introduction

What Is Intermittent Fasting?

Intermittent fasting can be described as alternating intervals of feeding periods and not eating (fasting) period. It simply means you alternate a feeding window and a fasting window. The length of time for each window will vary heavily depending on the protocol of fasting you adopt.

Your body is structured for a smooth transition between fasted and fed states. When in the fed state the level of insulin is elevated thereby signaling the body to store all excess calories in fat cells. The burning of fat is also halted and the body burns the glucose from your previous meal instead. On the other hand, when your body is in the fasted state insulin levels drop and hormones that oppose insulin (growth and glucagon hormones) are elevated. This forces the body to burn fat stored in the fat cells to produce energy. This simply means burning fat can only happen when the body is in the fasted state and store more fat when in the fed state.

The moment you begin eating your body enters into the fed state, for the next 3-5 hours the works on the food you consume. The level of insulin in your body rises significantly thereby shutting off fat burning and storing the excess calories. After the mentioned hours the body will enter the post-absorptive state. In the absorptive state, the body is still circulating the components from the last meal you ate. The post absorptive state last for 8-12 hours after the last meal taken. It takes 12 hours for your body to fully go into the fasted state.

The idea behind intermittent fasting is eating ad libitum when the feeding window opens and when the fasting window starts you avoid drinking or eating stuff with caloric value, but tea or coffee sweetened with erythritol or stevia are allowed. What this means is eating to satiety without compromising your daily macronutrients levels.

You might be new to the concept of intermittent fasting, but you have practiced a form of fasting before. The difference is that in most cases you fast haphazardly i.e. you do not follow a structured fasting timetable, and for this reason, you end up gaining no benefit.

For example, sleeping can be described as a fasting window. When you are sleeping you practice a fairly rigid period of fasting which can last for 6-8 hours per night before you take your breakfast. This is the reason your first meal for the day is called breakfast (breaking your overnight fast).

By nature, intermittent fasting is intermittent and is no way remotely similar to anorexia. This is because IF is done for controlled periods which are brief whereas anorexia an extreme caloric restriction sustained with a goal to lose fat extremely fast. One of the best examples of intermittent fasting is Ramadan; practiced for 4 weeks by Muslims.

The History of Fasting

As I'm sure you're well aware, fasting has been and continued to be a part of our world. From various religious fasts still observed today (Ramadan and Yom Kippur, for example) to starvation protests, we see how depriving the body of food can be used. While starvation protests don't exactly lead to healthier bodies, in most cases, they do make a dramatic point about the greater needs of a person or a group of people that can't be met through food.

Religions have used fasting as a way to clear the mind, purify the body, and help the soul reach out to the preferred greater power. This in itself is interesting when we look at the scientific benefits of fasting — Buddhist monks, for example, are renowned for their amazing and almost supernatural abilities. The monks employ fasting as a regular part of their lives as a method to practice self-control. If this concept interests you, do some research into various religious fasting practices to see what use they are put to and how science currently proves or disproves those theories.

Secularly, we can see a history of fasting in the way in which humans survived. In ancient times, we were hunters and gatherers, and therefore most of our meals were not guaranteed or expected. We searched for food, and when we found none, we starved. Our bodies, genetically than, are conditioned to go without food for a long period and then potentially feast after. This is why scientists suppose that our bodies have increased reaction and sensitivity to food after a fasting period — it's not just because our bodies need fuel, now! It's also because we need be able to work harder to find that food. We need to be able to act quickly and think clearer to survive. Thus, our bodies adapt and provide us with the ability to do so through improved norepinephrine and epinephrine production — when fasting, we adapt to increase our adrenaline output to be more efficient hunter-gatherers. Now that's food for thought!

So, if we are conditioned to fast already, why isn't it easier? We have worked very hard as a species to ensure our hunting and gathering limits are within 100m of our homes. Most of us no longer have to work very hard for our sustenance. On top of that, most people don't willingly put themselves into uncomfortable situations like fasting. However, perhaps this is also adding to the obesity epidemic we see in the modern world where there is no lack of or struggle for food. With that in mind, perhaps going back to our roots and re-introducing some level of fasting is beneficial to us for our bodies and our minds. Keep a journal of your progress as you fast and note your mental clarity each day of your fasts — what improvements do you see over time, if any?

While fasting in the health and wellness world for weight loss is fairly new to the scene, despite ages of the history of fasting, we can still see back about 80 years to when fasting for health improvement started emerging. There have been various champions for the fasting movement recently, such as Martin Berkhan in about 2010 when he created Leangains (a style of intermittent fasting) and Brad Pilon who created Eat-Stop-Eat (a type of alternate day fasting) around the same time. This is an exciting time for dietary science because we can finally study the effects of all types of fasting on the body and see if any of our history of fasting can be rationalized with science, and to what extent.

Intermittent Fasting for Women

For women who are interested in weight loss, intermittent fasting may seem like

a great choice, but many people want to know, should women fast? Is intermittent fasting effective for women? There have been a few critical studies about intermittent fasting which can help to shed some light on this interesting new dietary trend.

Intermittent fasting is also known as alternate-day fasting, although there are certainly some variations on this diet. The American Journal of Clinical Nutrition performed a study recently that enrolled 16 obese men and women in a 10-week program. On the fasting days, participants consumed food to 25% of their estimated energy needs. The rest of the time, they received dietary counseling but were not given a specific guideline to follow during this time.

As expected, the participants lost weight due to this study, but what researchers found interesting were some specific changes. The subjects were all still obese after just 10 weeks, but they had shown improvement in cholesterol, LDL-cholesterol, triglycerides, and systolic blood pressure. What made this an interesting find was that most people have to lose more weight than these study participants before seeing the same changes. It was a fascinating discovery which has spurred a significant number of individuals to try fasting.

Intermittent fasting for women has some beneficial effects. What makes it especially important for women who are trying to lose weight is that women have a much higher large proportion in their bodies. When trying to lose weight, the body primarily burns through carbohydrate stores with the first 6 hours and then starts to burn fat. Women who are following a healthy diet and exercise plan may be struggling with stubborn fat, but fasting is a realistic solution to this.

Intermittent Fasting For Women Over 50

Apparently, our bodies and our metabolism change when we hit menopause. One of the biggest changes that women over 50 experiences is that they have a slower metabolism and they start to put on weight. Fasting may be a good way to reverse and prevent this weight gain though. Studies have shown that this fasting pattern helps to regulate appetite and people who follow it regularly do not experience the same cravings that others do. If you're over 50 and trying to adjust to your slower metabolism, intermittent fasting can help you to avoid eating too much on a daily basis.

When you reach 50, your body also starts to develop some chronic diseases like high cholesterol and high blood pressure. Intermittent fasting has been shown to decrease both cholesterol and blood pressure, even without a large amount of weight loss. If you've started to notice your numbers rising at the doctor's office each year, you may be able to bring them back down with fasting, even without losing much weight.

Intermittent fasting may not be a splendid idea for every woman. Anyone with a particular health condition or who tends to be hypoglycemic should consult with a doctor. However, this new dietary trend has specific benefits for women who naturally store more fat in their bodies and may have trouble getting rid of these fat stores.

How To Quickly Lose Fat For Women

Losing fat can be very simple, but at the same time, it can be very frustrating. It's simple because weight loss is not a complicated equation. As long as you are consuming fewer calories than what your body burns you will lose weight. On the flipside, this can be very frustrating for those who don't know how to create the caloric deficit needed without depriving or starving themselves. Whatever the reason for wanting to lose weight, we are ultimately racing against time. So, here are the best ways to quickly lose fat for women.

Intermittent Fasting For Fat Loss

The fitness industry has given fasting for weight loss a bad rap over the past few years. There have been a lot of misconceptions and myths around fasting that people seem to get nervous about the idea. Let's first address the myths before we can move forward. Fasting does not cause your body to go into the infamous "starvation mode," nor does it slow the metabolism or breakdown muscle. The fitness industry has us believe that we have to regularly eat small meals throughout the day to keep the metabolism going. If we skip a meal or miss breakfast, our body goes into starvation mode which somehow causes the metabolism to slow down. It is one of the biggest myths in the industry.

The Wonderful Benefits Of Intermittent Fasting For Women

The pattern of eating called "Intermittent Fasting" usually means one fast for a period and eats for a period. Many choose a 24-hour cycle of fasting, then eat healthy the next day, and continue this process as a lifestyle change.

Research has been done on animals to find the benefits of this type of fasting, and you will be happy to know it really can be beneficial to your health!

Intermittent fasting can add 40%-56% more years to your life! That in itself is reason enough to do it. However other benefits include body weight reduction and fat oxidation.

When you fast, your body is forced to scavenge for fuel thus removing aged and damaged cells in the process. It cleanses the body of annoying and unwanted things and helps the weight loss and benefits of the healthy food choices be increased and more beneficial to your body.

Rats have been shown to have long-term and improved survival after heart failure after being on an IF eating plan, too. Researchers are also saying that it might help age-related deficits in cognitive function, too, so that tells me that it might help ward off Alzheimer's Disease and other types of Dementia!
Your risk of heart disease and other heart ailments may also be decreased when you start a healthy intermittent fasting regimen. Your risk for other chronic illnesses and diseases will also most likely be reduced.

A healthier you can begin with intermittent fasting and healthy food choices! Keep carbs to 50-100 grams per day. Many women eat between 1200-1500 calories per day, and when limiting their carbs, they are still

losing weight. Of course, less is best, and you need to determine caloric intake based on your activity such as working hard and exercising.

Drinking Lots of Fluids

Drink lots of fluids, especially water and exercise in the evenings if possible. It will help with that late-night cravings.

Once you start eating and drinking healthier, your body won't crave as much (if any) junk food, so making healthy food choices will simply get easier and easier as you progress in the intermittent fasting routine.

Alternate Day Fasting or ADF means alternating days of eating and not eating any food, but there is also an intermittent fasting called Modified Fasting where you consume about 20% of your normal calories one day and then eat regularly (but healthy) the next day. It is often more attainable for people because they feel less deprived when they can at least eat something daily, and it still has most of the benefits of the ADF regimen.

Whatever you choose to do, make sure you tell your health care professional of your plans so he or she is aware and can work with you to reach your goals. If you want to lose weight, lose fat and feel better, then intermittent fasting might be the answer for you!

To sum things up, you really can attain a feminine, firm, fit and younger appearance regardless of your age or inherited traits. You can overcome any weaknesses and trouble spots to some extent with balanced and symmetrical strength, cardiovascular and flexibility training, combined with making nutritious food choices.

Focus on being the best you can be. A lean and healthy body is both realistic and achievable.

Where to Start?

Incorporate fasting into daily schedule
For fasting to work for you, you have to be consistent with your method of choice. The easiest way is to make intermittent fast a lifestyle. Below are some tips to help you with it:
Starting process

- Drink 3 cups of water in the morning
- Plan your meal for the end of the fast
- Check your body fitness to see if you will add supplements if you are pregnant
- Take a cup of coffee
- Hit the gym if you are fasting for weight loss

During the day

- Take 2 cups of water for lunch
- Take a nap in the afternoons if you are at home
- Don't forget your sugar-free gum
- You can visit friends or catch up on reading

After the fast

- Prepare your meal for breaking the fast
- Always measure your calorie intake
- Drink 3 cups few minutes before you break your fast
- Take your meal
- Take a long nap

The dos and don'ts of fasting

Fasting is good, and many people have been practicing this for a long time now. Some people do it unknowingly by skipping breakfast while some have been doing it for religious purposes. However, no matter your reason for fasting, make sure to observe some of the rules to fasting.

Dos

- Fast when you are fit. Avoid fasting when you are pregnant, lactating or sick and under treatment.
- Make your fast part of your lifestyle. Integrate fasting into your daily routine for consistency
- Make sure your mind and body is prepared for the fast. Change your thought process by seeing fasting as a health practice instead of deprivation
- Prepare your kitchen by shopping for the right foods. Let your kitchen contain the right kinds of foods so that you don't consume junk after fasting
- Engage in light exercise, not heavy lifting so as not to break down
- Take enough vitamins to serve as back up to the light meals you eat
- Get a fast friend. This will encourage you to do better
- Distract yourself with fun stuff. You don't have to be morose or appear sickly. You don't need a pity party.

Don'ts

- Don't forget to tell your doctor about your intermittent fasting schedule. S/he might change your medication, adjust its dosage or timing to sync with your fasting schedule.

- Avoid stress
- Don't eat a lot for your last meal before the fast. Make sure your diet includes lean protein, vegetables and fats only.
- Don't ignore the importance of water during fasting. Drink encugh of it to stay hydrated at all time
- Don't push yourself too hard. You don't need to impress anybody nor be a hero. You are doing it for yourself
- Don't celebrate the end of fasting or you will go back to accumulating more fats than you burnt

Why Intermittent Fasting?

In the world today, there are numerous ways that you can use to lose weight. But, why should you choose intermittent fasting over all those others?

This chapter is going to show you why intermittent fasting stands out among other weight loss methods by highlighting the various benefits that come with it as it is more than just a weight loss program. Some benefits you stand to gain by practicing intermittent fasting are as follows.

Better Detoxification

This may come to you as a surprise, but your body cleanses and detoxifies itself on a daily basis. Millions of cellular processes go on in your body, and it is usually your body's duty to identify the worn-out cells and replace them. This process is commonly known as autophagy, and it is a normal process that happens constantly.

The ongoing process of autophagy is usually affected by two things. The first one is a bad diet, and the second one is frequent eating. Usually, when you eat, the process of autophagy is slowed down because your body changes its focus from cleansing and detoxifying to digestion and absorption.

If you take meals only a few hours (5–6 hours) apart from each other, your cleansing process normally slows down making you feel tired as the lack of repair will be taking a toll on your cells.
One of the advantages of intermittent fasting is that it gives your body time to focus on the process of cellular repair because it discourages constant eating and encourages long hours of fasting. Therefore, with intermittent fasting, you stand a chance of boosting your body's detoxification process.

Less Hunger

Intermittent fasting is considered one of the best ways to lose weight because it deals with the one thing that makes it difficult for people to follow a diet, hunger.

Intermittent fasting is known for managing hunger and appetite, which makes the process of losing weight easier and fun. But how does it do this? Intense hunger is usually caused by blood sugar fluctuations, especially when your diet is high in carbohydrates.

When you eat a high-carb meal, your body produces high levels of insulin to manage the sugar levels. Insulin encourages your body cells to use the energy, and the rest is stored as fat, and this leads to a sudden drop in blood sugar levels. This sends a message to your brain that you need to eat to maintain your blood sugar level and the cycle continues.

Intermitted fasting manages your appetite by controlling your hunger hormones. When you practice intermittent fasting, your body normally relies on stored fat for energy. When that happens, the fat cell produces a hormone called Leptin, which regulates the hunger hormone ghrelin. It does this by telling your brain to turn off the hunger signals from ghrelin, which makes you rarely feel hungry when you are fasting.

Lowered Risk of Type-2 Diabetes

One of the advantages of intermittent fasting is that it uses up all of the glucose in your body and starts using fat for energy. That process usually lowers your body's blood sugar levels, which in turn reduces your risk of getting type-2 diabetes.

According to a study that was done on intermittent fasting, it was found out that the blood sugar of a person practicing intermittent fasting reduced 3–6% while their insulin reduced by 20–31%. You can find this study here.

Reduced Oxidative Stress

Oxidative stress normally happens when your body has a higher production of free radicals than normal: free radicals include reactive oxygen species. Poorly functioning mitochondria normally cause these unstable molecules. Such molecules carry reactive electrons, which either take an electron or give up an electron when they encounter other molecules.

When that happens, the result is usually a fast chain reaction from one molecule to the other. That then ends up creating more of these free radicals that causes the connections between atoms in the DNA, cellular membrane, and the essential proteins to break apart and destroy. These damages not only stress your body out but also affects your ageing process since your cells are constantly being damaged.

What intermittent fasting does is that it lowers your blood sugar levels, which automatically forces your cells to turn to a survival process. When this happens, the cells quickly remove any mitochondria that are unhealthy and substitute them with new ones that are healthy as time goes on. This activity is the one that reduces the production of free radicals, which translates to a reduction in oxidative stress.

Reduced Risk of Cancer

The relationship between intermittent fasting and cancer has been heavily debated upon up to date. Some people suggest that intermittent fasting reduces the risk of cancer while others believe that more research needs to be done. But if this research is anything to go by, then intermittent fasting can help you reduce the risk of cancer.
The study consisted of 10 cancer patients. Half of them were subjected to intermittent fasting before going for a chemotherapy session while the other half were not. After the two groups went for chemotherapy, it was discovered that the cancer patients who practiced intermittent fasting experienced reduced side effects and even had better cure rates than their counterparts did.

Cancer is usually caused by uncontrolled growth of cells, which mainly depend on the energy that comes from glucose to grow. Therefore, when you fast, you cut the energy channel that the cells need to grow. This causes the abnormal cells to stop growing completely or slow down.
Longevity

One of the most sort-after benefits of intermittent fasting is its ability to help you live a longer life. Numerous studies in rats have proven that intermittent fasting can extend your life span. In one of the rat studies, it was seen that rats that fasted daily lived 83% longer than those ones that didn't fast.

Now that you know how you can benefit from intermittent fasting, the next step is for you to find out how you can start practicing intermittent fasting and the methods that you will be using.

Types of Intermittent Fasting

Intermittent fasting has become very trendy in the past few years, and several different types/methods have emerged.

Here are some of the most popular ones:

The 16/8 Method: Fast for 16 hours each day, for example by only eating between noon and 8pm.

Eat-Stop-Eat: Once or twice a week, don't eat anything from dinner one day, until dinner the next day (a 24 hour fast).
The 5:2 Diet: During 2 days of the week, eat only about 500-600 calories.

Then there are many other variations.

I am personally a fan of the 16/8 method (popularized by Martin Berkhan of LeanGains), as I find it to be the simplest and the easiest to stick with.

In fact, I pretty much naturally eat this way. I am usually not very hungry in the morning, and don't feel compelled to eat until about 1 pm. Then I eat my last meal somewhere between 6-9pm, so I end up instinctively fasting for 16-19 hours every day.

Bottom Line: There are many different intermittent fasting methods. The most popular ones are the 16/8 method, Eat-Stop-Eat and the 5:2 diet.
Take Home Message

As long as you stick to healthy foods, restricting your eating window and fasting from time to time, you can have some very impressive health benefits.

It is an effective way to lose fat and improve metabolic health, while simplifying your life at the same time.

Popular Ways to do Intermittent Fasting:

1. The 16/8 Method: Fast for 16 hours each day

The 16/8 Method involves fasting every day for 14-16 hours, and restricting your daily "eating window" to 8-10 hours. Within the eating window, you can fit in 2, 3 or more meals.

This method is also known as the Leangains protocol, and was popularized by fitness expert Martin Berkhan. Doing this method of fasting can actually be as simple as not eating anything after dinner, and skipping breakfast.

For example, if you finish your last meal at 8 pm and then don't eat until 12 noon the next day, then you are technically fasting for 16 hours between meals.

It is generally recommended that women only fast 14-15 hours, because they seem to do better with slightly shorter fasts. For people who get hungry in the morning and like to eat breakfast, then this can be hard to get used to at first. However, many breakfast skippers actually instinctively eat this way. You can drink water, coffee and other non-caloric beverages during the fast, and this can help reduce hunger levels.

It is very important to eat mostly healthy foods during your eating window. This won't work if you eat lots of junk food or excessive amounts of calories.

I find this to be the most "natural" way to do intermittent fasting. I eat this way myself and find it to be 100% effortless.

I eat a low-carb diet, so my appetite is blunted somewhat. I simply do not feel hungry until around 1 pm in the afternoon. Then I eat my last meal around 6-9 pm, so I end up fasting for 16-19 hours.

Bottom Line: The 16/8 method involves daily fasts of 16 hours for men, and 14-15 hours for women. On each day, you restrict your eating to an 8-10 hour "eating window" where you can fit in 2-3 or more meals.

2. The 5:2 Diet: Fast for 2 days per week

The 5:2 diet involves eating normally 5 days of the week, while restricting calories to 500-600 on two days of the week. This diet is also called the Fast diet, and was popularized by British journalist and doctor Michael Mosley. On the fasting days, it is recommended that women eat 500 calories, and men 600 calories.

For example, you might normally eat on all days except Mondays and Thursdays, where you eat two small meals (250 calories per meal for women, and 300 for men). As critics correctly point out, there are no studies testing the 5:2 diet itself, but there are plenty of studies on the benefits of intermittent fasting.

Bottom Line: The 5:2 diet, or the Fast diet, involves eating 500-600 calories for two days of the week but eating normally the other 5 days.

3. Eat-Stop-Eat: Do a 24-hour fast, once or twice a week

Eat-Stop-Eat involves a 24-hour fast, either once or twice per week. This method was popularized by fitness expert Brad Pilon, and has been quite popular for a few years.

By fasting from dinner one day, to dinner the next, this amounts to a 24-hour fast.

For example, if you finish dinner on Monday at 7 pm, and don't eat until dinner the next day at 7 pm, then you've just done a full 24-hour fast. You can also fast from breakfast to breakfast, or lunch to lunch. The end result is the same. Water, coffee and other non-caloric beverages are allowed during the fast, but no solid food.

If you are doing this to lose weight, then it is very important that you eat normally during the eating periods. As in, eat the same amount of food as if you hadn't been fasting at all.

The problem with this method is that a full 24-hour fast can be fairly difficult for many people.

However, you don't need to go all-in right away, starting with 14-16 hours and then moving upwards from there is fine. I've personally done this a few times. I found the first part of the fast very easy, but in the last few hours I did become ravenously hungry.

I needed to apply some serious self-discipline to finish the full 24-hours and often found myself giving up and eating dinner a bit earlier.

Bottom Line: Eat-Stop-Eat is an intermittent fasting program with one or two 24-hour fasts per weeks.

4. Alternate-Day Fasting: Fast every other day

Alternate-Day fasting means fasting every other day. There are several different versions of this. Some of them allow about 500 calories during the fasting days. Many of the lab studies showing health benefits of intermittent fasting used some version of this. A full fast every other day seems rather extreme, so I do not recommend this for beginners. With this method, you will be going to bed very hungry several times per week, which is not very pleasant and probably unsustainable in the long-term.

Bottom Line: Alternate-day fasting means fasting every other day, either by not eating anything or only eating a few hundred calories.

5. The Warrior Diet: Fast during the day, eat a huge meal at night

The Warrior Diet was popularized by fitness expert Ori Hofmekler. It involves eating small amounts of raw fruits and vegetables during the day, then eating one huge meal at night.

Basically, you "fast" all day and "feast" at night within a 4 hour eating window. The Warrior Diet was one of the first popular "diets" to include a form of intermittent fasting. This diet also emphasizes food choices that are quite similar to a paleo diet – whole, unprocessed foods that resemble what they looked like in nature.

Bottom Line: The Warrior Diet is about eating only small amounts of vegetables and fruits during the day, then eating one huge meal at night.

6. Spontaneous Meal Skipping: Skip meals when convenient

You don't need to follow a structured intermittent fasting plan to reap some of the benefits. Another option is to simply skip meals from time to time, when you don't feel hungry or are too busy to cook and eat. It's a myth that people need to eat every few hours, or they will hit "starvation mode" or lose muscle. The human body is well equipped to handle long periods of famine, let alone missing one or two meals from time to time.

So if you're not hungry one day, skip breakfast and just eat a healthy lunch and dinner. Or if you're traveling and can't find anything you want to eat, do a short fast.

Skipping 1 or 2 meals when, you feel so inclined is basically a spontaneous intermittent fast. Just make sure to eat healthy foods at the other meals.

Bottom Line: Another more "natural" way to do intermittent fasting is to simply skip 1 or 2 meals when you don't feel hungry or don't have time to eat.

Take Home Message

There are a lot of people getting great results with some of these methods.

That being said, if you're already happy with your health and don't see much room for improvement, then feel free to safely ignore all of this. Intermittent fasting is not for everyone. It is not something that anyone needs to do, it is just another tool in the toolbox that can be useful for some people. Some also believe that it may not be as beneficial for women as men, and it may also be a poor choice for people who are prone to eating disorders. If you decide to try this out, then keep in mind that you need to eat healthy as well. It is not possible to binge on junk foods during the eating periods and expect to lose weight and improve health.

Calories still count, and food quality is still absolutely crucial.

What Can I Expect from Intermittent Fasting?

One of the main questions I get, when it comes to intermittent fasting is, "What can I expect?". This might mean, what do I expect during fasting and it might be about what effects one might achieve from fasting, or it might be both. In this chapter, we will cover what you might expect during fasting and what kind of results you might expect to achieve.

You should keep in mind that everyone's body is different and the way in which people's bodies metabolize foods may vary quite a bit from person to person. Therefore, you should understand that there is no set "what to expect" when it comes to intermittent fasting. I can tell you some things you might experience while fasting and what the end results might be, but I can't tell you definitively what you can expect from it.

During the fast

Of course, one thing you should expect when you first start fasting is you are going to be hungry. While I know this should go without saying, I have found quite a few people who were genuinely surprised at how hungry they were while fasting (especially with 24+ hour fasting). Many tell me that, although they expected to feel some hunger, they never expected to feel THAT hungry. While some may only experience mild hunger that passes, most do experience extreme hunger when they first start fasting. The good news is that the more you stick with your fasting regime, the easier it does become and after a while, the hunger is almost unnoticeable. A good way to stave off hunger is to drink plenty of water. Not only does water keep you hydrated (which is very important while fasting) but it also makes you feel fuller.

If the hunger is too much for you to handle, however, you might want to try to lower your actual fasting time. For instance, if you can go 4 hours without feeling any hunger, then another 2 before feeling like you will die if you don't get something to eat, then set your fasting window at about 5-6 hours. Do this for a week or so, then try increasing the window to see how long you can go. However, I would suggest that you try to go as long as you can, even if you are extremely hungry. Sometimes, the hunger passes as your body begins to metabolize the fatty acids in your system and starts producing more energy.

Speaking of energy, that's another question I get asked all the time about intermittent fasting, "Will my energy level increase or decrease while fasting, or will it stay about the same?". Again, it depends on quite a bit on what kind of metabolism you have. If you normally have a very slow metabolism, you will more than likely see an increase in energy while fasting as your metabolism will speed up from fasting. On the other hand, if you have a very fast metabolism, you may not notice any energy difference between fasting and non-fasting periods. If you do notice anything, it may be a slight decrease in energy, but then that would be only temporarily. Even if you do have a slow metabolism, sometimes people still fill a lack of energy during their fasting periods. This may be due to a lack of key vitamins or other nutrients in your system. If you feel extremely lethargic during fasting, it would be a good idea to see your doctor or other health practitioners.

Intermittent fasting is especially helpful for those with a slow metabolism, as it inevitably causes your metabolism to speed up, even during non-fasting days. It's kind of like training for running. When you first start training, you may not be able to run very fast, but as you continue to run, your speed increases exponentially. When you fast, your metabolism is forced to kick it up a notch. The more your metabolism increases during fasting, the more it also increases during normal eating periods as it is learning to process foods more sensibly.

Some other things you may experience during your first few periods of intermittent fasting include dizziness, lethargy, weakness, nervousness and/or anxiety, irritability, headaches, and problems sleeping. These are some of the more commonly reported side effects, though you may never experience any of them at all. The good news is, most of these side effects are mild and usually disappear after a few more periods of fasting. If any of these symptoms, however, are severe or persistent you would do very well to see a health practitioner as soon as possible, as there may be an underlying condition.

How much weight can I lose and how fast?

Another very popular question is "I know intermittent fasting is supposed to help me lose weight, but how much weight can I expect to lose and how fast?". Well, I don't mean to sound like a broken record but... again, this varies widely from person to person. Some have found a very rapid weight loss, with intermittent fasting, while others only noticed any significant weight loss over a long period. The average person probably fits somewhere between these extremes.

It also depends on quite a bit on the method of intermittent fasting you are using. Of course, the longer your fasting periods are, the more rapidly your weight will come off. The main point of losing weight through intermittent fasting is to keep your calories in deficit. This means you need to burn more calories than you consume. When you consume 0 calories for 24 hours, you should automatically go into deficit mode... even if all you did was sleep, your body is still using calories for basic functions such as breathing and maintaining a proper body temperature.

While it may be true you can burn calories while doing nothing; you will find it takes much longer than if you simply get active. If you have a sedentary lifestyle, you will find your metabolism is extremely low, and you will find yourself easily fatigued from even the most basic activities, such as walking, housecleaning, washing the car or doing the laundry. The problem with many people who have a low metabolism is that they find it very difficult to get out and walk or run and exercise regularly... they are simply too fatigued to start being active. Intermittent fasting will help you in this, as you will more than likely have a bit more energy after a few periods of fasting. You will be able to take advantage of that extra energy by exercising, maybe bicycling or running, even do some aerobics. By constructively utilizing that extra energy, you will burn much more calories while fasting and even start burning more calories during non-fasting periods.

To keep it simple, if you want to lose weight, you MUST burn more calories than you consume. Most diet pills, shakes, etc. are designed to help you burn those calories faster, but most of these concoctions are not good for you and may even be quite deleterious to your health and well-being. You are much better off with intermittent fasting than any diet pill on the market. Intermittent fasting is much safer and has been around longer than any of those concoctions have. Fasting has a great track record, and it's safe and effective.

If you have an average metabolism and fast 24 hours, 3 days a week, you should start seeing anywhere from 3-5 pounds (or more) of weight loss per week. Of course, one of the highest determining factors of how much weight you might lose is how much food you consume during non-fasting periods. You should try to keep your calories consistent and not gorge on food during your non-fasting periods. Also, you should try to get as much fiber and protein as you can.

If you regularly work out, such as weight lifting and other muscle building exercises, you may see less weight loss as the fat is being converted into muscle, rather than it being burned off and converted into energy. You should still see some weight loss, but if you want to really build your muscles you want to keep your calories in surplus, so that your body can utilize those extra calories for muscles, which means you should eat more during windows of non-fasting while working out so that there are plenty of calories to burn and turn into muscles.

If you are fasting intermittently and still not seeing any pounds coming off, there may be a few reasons why. The first, and most obvious reasons would be you don't have enough fat to burn; you are already at your "best" weight. You will still find intermittent fasting as goo method for keeping your weight at the ideal point as well as keeping you energized. On the other hand, if you are obviously overweight, then the problem may very well be what you are eating during non-fasting periods. If you are eating fewer calories than you consume, then you

should be losing weight. But, if you are eating junk foods, foods high in cholesterol and high in fat content, you may be making more fat than you are burning, especially if you gorge on these foods right before your fasting period.

Intermittent fasting can help you lose weight, but you need to make the conscious decision to eat right and to keep a healthy diet if you want to see dramatic results from intermittent fasting. We have included, toward the end of this book, a few different ideas for a good diet between you fasting periods. These plans are based on a standard 16-hour fasting plan (which means you have an 8-hour window of eating). These plans are based on a 1600 calorie intake, but you may require less or more depending on your body type and your metabolic rate.

Can't I eat whatever I want during my eating window?

You can eat almost anything during non-fasting periods and still (possibly) see positive results from intermittent fasting. If you want to see those results quickly and make it much easier on yourself, however you should plan your meals during those non-fasting periods. You should plan to make healthy decisions, such as whole grains, fresh fruits and vegetables, lean meat (if you like to eat meat) and generally foods high in protein, avoiding most starchy foods (though resistant starches are good) and foods that have high calories but low nutritional values (also known as empty calories).

It doesn't take that long to sit down and plan on healthy meals, and it makes it much easier on your system when you do fast. If you consume too much junk while not fasting, your body is going to have a deficit of proteins to draw on during the fasting periods, and most of the calories have already been turned into fat, thus requiring the body to take most of its energy from fat to burn more fat, which means it will take it much longer to burn away those fat calories.

Take your time to examine these plans, then adapt them toward your likes. You will find that by just taking the time to plan out your meals, you will be more prone to choosing those foods that are better for you. If you very rarely plan your meals, you may find it a chore at first, but after a while, it becomes a fun activity as you find yourself looking forward to those meals and knowing exactly what you are going to be eating. As you begin to eat healthier foods, you will begin to see an increase in your energy levels both during and after a fasting period; you will begin to enjoy activities that you might have put on a back shelf, due to low energy.

What I'm saying is yes, intermittent fasting does allow you to eat whatever you like during non-fasting periods as this is not a diet, but more of a lifestyle change... but at the same time – if you eat healthier meals during non-fasting periods, then intermittent fasting will help you much more and much more rapidly. You will notice a much more dramatic change in your energy levels and your overall well-being if you simply make a few changes in your diet to allow for more nutrients, vitamins, minerals and the like.

Specific Considerations When Implementing Intermittent Fasting

You've now got a thorough understanding of the background of intermittent fasting, the scientifically based evidence of its benefits, how to do it, and how to work this cycle of eating into your life.

There are some considerations as to who may or may not benefit from intermittent fasting. There are a lot of women (and men) who have gotten great weight loss results using some form of fasting and cycled eating. However, just like any diet and exercise program or regimen, intermittent fasting is not for everyone, and it's important you practice the proper weight loss plan for your body and your specific goals. Intermittent fasting is certainly not something that everyone needs to do, but it's a helpful tool in the weight loss battle that so many women struggle with. It can be easily implemented in many women's daily lives and used to promote greater overall health and well-being, but it can, in some cases, be misused as well.

There are a few pre-requisites that if followed, will make your intermittent fasting weight loss journey easier and more successful, and make you a good candidate for reaping the most benefits from this program. These include the following:

• Get enough sleep on a regular basis.

• Minimize stress in your daily life.

• Make sure lifestyle activity is within a normal range—not too much or too little daily movement and exercise.

• Be fat adapted. This means that your body can easily access and burn stored fat throughout the day when it's needed to provide energy.

So, how can you tell if you're already considered fat adapted? No blood test can give you this answer, but there are a few simple questions you can ask yourself that should be able to provide you with an indication of your level of fat adaptability:

• Can you go 3 hours or more without eating? Would skipping a meal be an incredibly difficult physical and mental struggle for you?

• On a normal day, do you feel your energy level stays consistent throughout the day? Do you need to take an afternoon nap or is it just something you enjoy doing now and again?

• Are you able to perform a fairly vigorous physical activity like steady walking, jogging, or light exercise without first consuming carbohydrates for energy?

• Do you frequently suffer from headaches, mental exhaustion, and mental fog?

Someone whose body is fat adapted can usually skip meals with little effort on their part. They have consistent energy and do not require an afternoon nap to make it through the second portion of their day. They can be moderately active and perform physical activities like brisk walking, jogging, hiking, biking, and swimming without needing to fuel their body beforehand with carbohydrates, and they do not suffer from the mental fog, headaches, and exhaustion that a person whose body is more sugar dependent may.

Some of you are lucky and are genetically predisposed to be a fat burning machine! Others of you may not be, and your genetics may require more effort than the first group to reach this state of fat burning and freedom from sugar and carbohydrate dependence. Luckily for all of us, your genes are not final! They don't define you, and they can be altered! Through your behavior and your lifestyle choices, you have the ability to turn on and off various genes in your genetic code that can lead to the physical results you desire. There are numerous versions of the future person you may become, and it's always up to you to make the decisions that will ultimately lead to who you will become. You are responsible for making choices and living a lifestyle that will promote and direct your genes toward fat loss, building muscle, and overall wellness. Following an intermittent fasting style of eating will put you on the path to achieving this longevity of life and general wellness of the body.

If you feel that you may be lacking in the fat-adaptability department and want to give yourself the best start to your intermittent fasting protocol, it can benefit you to try eating the paleo style diet for 3 weeks before beginning your cycles of fasting and eating. This means you'll eliminate sugar, grains, legumes, and vegetable oils from your diet for 3 weeks before beginning intermittent fasting. This should be the push your body needs to become more efficient in drawing upon fat stores for energy rather than relying on dietary sugar for fuel. Again, this step is not necessary for your pursuit of weight loss through intermittent fasting, but it can set you up for the most success in the shortest possible time.

Are there any indicators of someone whom intermittent fasting may not be beneficial for?

Intermittent fasting may not be a great protocol to follow for someone who is susceptible to eating disorders. If you've had a problem with disordered eating at any point in your life, it might be beneficial for you to explore multiple weight loss plans before deciding what works best for you. If intermittent fasting seems like the best choice for your lifestyle, do take the time to pay special attention to the amount of food you're consuming when you are not in your fasting periods, just to be sure you do not continuously deny yourself nutrition.

Intermittent fasting is considered a stressor on your body systems. You're using planned fasting and hunger to ignite metabolic processes within your body that respond to these stressors. For this reason, someone with a multitude of other stressors may not fare as well while following an intermittent fasting protocol. Mental stress, physical stress, and emotional stress can all hinder your mental ability to properly complete your fasting cycles as well as your body's physical ability to lose weight. Adding this new stressor can compound any other existing stressors, which won't be the most effective way to begin your weight loss journey.

Intermittent fasting may not be beneficial for someone with a cortisol regulation disorder. If you're actively monitoring your cortisol levels with your doctor or if you think you may have an issue with cortisol regulation it would be best to seek a professional opinion before implementing a fast into your weight loss regimen. Fasting raises cortisol levels in the body, and in a healthy individual, this poses no threat or health issue. Someone with a cortisol dysregulation can have serious side effects if their levels become excessive, and an activity that boosts production of cortisol may not be right for these people. If you think you may have an issue with cortisol regulation, visit your doctor before starting a program and find out for sure. You may have an issue with cortisol regulation if you retain excess belly fat, consistently lack enough sleep, persistently suffer from low-grade stress, and rely on caffeine to keep you awake and energized each day.

Should a pregnant woman practice intermittent fasting?

There haven't been many studies done on the effects of fasting on pregnant women on their growing fetus. One study that followed pregnant women fasting for Ramadan showed that these women had a

decrease in the development and growth of their placentas, but the slower growth was more efficient. The developing fetus grew as normal, but the women had much smaller reserves of nutrients in their bodies. Although this (and a few other) studies show that short-term fasting is probably safe during pregnancy, it is most likely a better idea to wait until after giving birth. Fasting during pregnancy is not necessary (except in these cases of religiously required fasts) and is probably not beneficial to the woman or her growing baby.

Should I fast if I am a diabetic?

This is a gray area and should be reviewed with your doctor before you begin. Women have a more difficult time regulating their blood sugar than men and can be more severely affected by a drop in blood sugar. There have been accounts of men who were classified as diabetic using intermittent fasting to control their blood sugar levels, lose weight, and effectively beat type-2 diabetes, but there have been no such accounts for women.

Will intermittent fasting affect my menstrual cycle and fertility? Humans are highly biologically effective at adapting to their environments. When proper nutrition is not available, it is more work for a woman's body to create new life and provide nutrition for the baby once it's born. For this reason, women are biologically designed to respond to the presence or scarcity of available food by altering some aspects of fertility. There haven't been clinical studies directly comparing the effects of intermittent fasting on female fertility. These studies do have to look at, mostly, and compare fertility changes due to extreme fasting circumstances like famine or anorexia—which are not truly comparable to planned and purposeful intermittent fasting. These studies do show a link between decreased fertility, the loss of a menstrual cycle, and fasting, but the differences between these scenarios and intermittent fasting should be considered. There is currently too little evidence-based clinical information on the relationship between intermittent fasting and female reproductive health to definitively say if it is beneficial, neutral, or harmful.

Do I Need to Change My Diet If I Use Intermittent Fasting?

I will begin by saying again that you should eat as healthily as you can – less processed junk, whole foods and plenty of green vegetables and water. However, you can be less than perfect with nutrition and still achieve results while fasting. It can be especially helpful to binge a little to keep sane – especially when trying something as demanding as fasting. Just don't consume more calories than you burn.

Onto the point though - intermittent fasting itself never requires a diet change by definition. Only a change in the times that you allow yourself to eat is necessary. Whether or not you choose to change your diet is up to you. Some people use IF purely for its health benefits. Others use it to prevent heart disease and diabetes. If you plan to lose weight and burn fat, however, you will need to change your diet in conjunction with IF.

The formula for weight loss is incredibly simple - so simple that it sounds almost too good to be true. All you need to do is take in less energy (calories) than you expend. That's it. It may sound easy, but in reality, it can be tough. Any health guru or fitness god who tells you that there's an easier way is quite simply lying and trying to sell you something. Sure, fat and nutrient macros are necessary if you are looking to maximize results and want a specific body fat percentage or maybe even if you're a bodybuilder. But if all you want to do is lose weight, energy (calories) is the only thing that matters. This is where IF comes in. Let's think of this mathematically.

To calculate how much energy (calories) you naturally spend without any exercise, you can use this formula:

655 + (4.35 × weight in lbs) + (4.7 × height in inches) – (4.7 × age)

If you are a 200 pound, 5' 5", a 27-year-old woman and you use Alternate Day Fasting (ADF)...

You expend 1,703 calories a day naturally, or 11,925 a week.

You take in 400 calories on your non-feeding days.

You take in 2,000 calories on your feeding days.

You take in 9,200 calories per week total.

That leaves an energy (calorie) deficit of 2,725 calories. A pound of fat is about 3,500 calories. That's almost a pound of fat lost per week with no exercise, and probably without even changing your eating habits that much on feeding days. You can imagine how much more you'd lose by eating a bit healthier and exercising on your non-feeding days.

If you are using IF without a diet change, you'll still reap significant health benefits (see the studies further up), but results won't be the absolute best. However, that doesn't mean that you can eat pizza and

cake on every feeding day. If you're a regular Sally and you eat sensibly, to begin with, your diet doesn't have to change dramatically

High-fat and low-fat diets have no effect on the health benefits of IF. This is one of the many reasons that IF is so popular these days. It's a simple, proven method for improving your health and extending your lifespan.

How Much Weight Can I Lose?

With intermittent fasting and a healthy lifestyle, you can lose any amount of weight you'd like. There's no limit! Okay, there is a limit to how much you can lose healthily. But, as long as you have a smaller amount of calories coming in than going out, you will lose weight. How quickly you lose that weight depends on how big the energy deficit is. To put it in simple terms, the more calories you lose, the more weight you lose. Easy! Actually, "how much weight can I lose" may be the wrong question to ask. The right question would be "how much weight should I lose, and how fast?" But first, let's cover an example.

There are about 3,500 calories in a pound of fat. Let's say that you want to lose 50 pounds. If you fast with a total calorie deficit of 3,500 calories a week - you will lose 1 pound per week or 50 pounds in 50 weeks. This is a safe, healthy amount of weight to lose in that period. Combine this with exercise, and you could lose an even larger amount of weight during this time while still maintaining your health. Intermittent fasting combined with exercise and a healthy diet is an easy and simple way to create that deficit naturally.

How much weight you should lose depends on your height. For reference, you should check with a BMI chart. The second half of the question, "how fast" is very important. Never attempt to lose more than 2 pounds a week.

Method 5:2 and 4:3

For this plan, you would eat a regular diet for five days. For the remaining two days, you will eat approximately 500 to 600 calories. The baseline of the calorie ingestion is 2,000 for women and 2,500 for men. A few famous names swear by the diet including Jennifer Aniston and David Cameron. These are some of the ways of how to manage the 5:2 diet plan; just remember carbs don't mix with your fasting days.

Experiment with Mealtime

- Test different eating times. It doesn't always have to be an early time of day when you aren't hungry. You can wait a bit longer if you wish.
- Change from eating three meals each day to two such as having brunch. It can combine the meals and save the calories. Try having brunch around 11 am and dinner at 7, or even a larger meal at 8 with your significant other.

Maximize the Flavoring and Minimize the Calories

- Soups are a respectable choice—also proven by research—because you remain full longer than just a modest serving of veggies on a plate.

- Flavor your foods with spices and herbs such as these—lemon juice or vinegar for salads or curry pastes or chili flakes in stews, baked beans, or soups.

- Go for the veggies and salads with smaller servings of fish, eggs, lean meat, or tofu.

Use Fresh Ingredients

- Not only are you eating better and healthier products, but also most fresh ingredients are less expensive. Search for seasonal produce for the most savings.

- Search for items such as a tomato that have ripened that would make a yummy treat with a few special herbs and balsamic vinegar. You could also add it to some soup.

- During the winter months, experiment with butternut squash or parsnip—roasted—with low-fat feta—or in soup.
- Cut some peppers in half and stuff them with cream cheese, tuna, or similar ingredients and grill them. You can add an egg to the mix for a taste challenge.

Food for the Fasting Days

- Berries and natural yogurt
- Plentiful veggie portions
- Baked or boiled eggs
- Low-cal 'cup' soups
- Other soups: vegetable, tomato, miso, cauliflower
- Lean mean or grilled fish
- Tea or black coffee

- Water (sparkling or still)

The 4:3 Diet Plan

Health benefits include asthma relief, reduction in heart arrhythmias, insulin resistance, menopausal hot flashes, seasonal allergies, and much more. After twelve weeks of fasting using the 4:3 method; these are the results from a small study group:

- Fat mass reduction: 3.5 kg with no muscle mass changes
- Body weight reduction: Over 5 kg
- Increased LDL particle size
- Reduced blood levels: 20% reduction of triglycerides
- Leptin levels: 40% decreased
- Levels CRP: Reduced levels (inflammation marker in your body)

How the 4:3 Diet Plan is Different from the 5:2 Plan

The 5:2 intermittent fasting choices are much simpler than the 4:3 plan because you are more restricted. You will be intermittently fasting for three out of the seven days. You should not eat processed/sugary/refined foods for four of the days. If you do, your body will crave the supplementary fatty acids you need to thrive.

If you consume junk on those four days, you will defeat the purpose of the plan. Just remember, not to over-indulge. As you train your body by eating a well-planned diet; your body will adjust to the routine, and you won't feel as hungry.

The 4:3 plan acclaims you skip the morning meal, and it recommends you check your weight daily. However, this can be disheartening if your weight fluctuates.

A sample plan for the 4:3 method of weight loss is as follows:

Breakfast: Eat nothing.

Lunch: Leek, lentil, or chicken soup with a snack such as a small tangerine

Dinner: A side salad using lemon juice as the dressing with some salt, pepper, or similar seasonings along with a small lean fillet of grilled chicken

Snacks: Veggies or fruit

You can have a light breakfast if you enjoy a morning meal, but you will need to eliminate the snack during the day. You can also skip lunch, and have a larger breakfast. This is more challenging to follow than the 5:2 intermittent fasting plan because you have three days you can only consume 500 calories versus two days on the 5:2 diet.

Suggestions for the Fasting Days Using the 4:3 Method

- Drink lots of water.
- Drink coffee and tea for additional boost.
- Consume a 400 calorie meal with a snack of 100 total calories.
- Chew sugar-free gum to fight the hunger spurts.

If you have a busy lifestyle, you can cheat once in a while with a low-calorie pre-packaged meal. (This is not a regular outlet.)

The point in both plans is to eat as much as you want and not feel deprived on the days you can eat normally—just do it in moderation, not over-indulgence.

The Lessons You Learn While Intermittent Fasting

Intermittent fasters have reported improved strength and leaner figures. The best part of this is that they didn't give up their favorite foods and feel cranky like they would have otherwise. While fasting, these same people have learned all sorts of lessons about the fasting process. They might provide a helpful guide to anyone that's getting started on the journey of intermittent fasting.

The biggest roadblock is your mind.

This diet, in comparison to all the other ones out there, is quite simple to implement into your life. Depending on how you have set up your fasting, you skip certain meals and make up for them at other meals. The biggest hurdle in this is telling your mind to accept the changes. People believe that if they aren't eating at particular times, they're going to faint or become ill or have some other adverse effects. People also believe that these particular times are roughly a couple hours apart. They also believe that skipping breakfast will ruin your day or that a light dinner will make them hungry during the night.

Starting fasting will help you realize how simple the diet is. People feel much healthier inside and out when they practice fasting. Many people find it best to ease into the diet instead of jumping in all at once. The lifestyle can go against everything that you were taught as children. You may even feel that it is adversely affecting your health to do something like this.   However, you will see how wrong you were once you see intermittent fasting in action.

Over time, you will find that your fears have no basis in the reality of the situation. You'll be healthier and more energetic than you were before you started intermittent fasting. The only thing you need to do is get yourself started on this journey.

You can easily lose weight and keep it off.

When you're consuming less calories than you burn, you lose weight. That's how weight lose works. Intermittent fasting is an easy method to this because it also avoids losing muscle mass. Those who need to lose weight for health reasons may turn to intermittent fasting because it doesn't mean much of a change in the diet that they had before intermittent fasting. The only change is when eating happens. Intermittent fasting works because when you eliminate meals and eat during your feeding time, there is a deficit of calories, assuming you don't completely binge.

Building muscle while fasting is extremely possible.
While using intermittent fasting, people report being able to gain lean muscle and cut off the fat by five percent. During the fasting period, your body is likely to lose weight. Because there is no steady flow of food and energy, your body will learn to turn to your fat stores and pull energy from there instead.

Because the fasts are short enough, your body won't turn to cannibalizing the muscles for energy. This means that there's little risk of losing muscle mass while practicing intermittent fasting. With eating, as long as you're consuming enough calories to build muscle, your body doesn't care when that food consumption happens. If it happens during an 8-hour period, the calories will affect you roughly the same as if you had eaten those calories over a 16-hour period or a 24-hour period.

Intermittent fasting can help your productivity.

While practicing intermittent fasting, many people report having improved mental clarity. This is especially true during the fasting periods. While we are told that fasting drains the body and mind of energy, this just isn't simply true. When the mind isn't focused so much on food, it can free up time for you to think about your other interests and hobbies.

Instead of thinking about dinner, you can think about a project that you've wanted to work on for a while. There's less time wasted when

you're making even one less meal a day. You don't have to shop, cook, wash, or spend time eating for that extra meal. You also don't have to worry about everything involved in it. The freed up time, and mental energy is great for getting on with projects and things that you want to get involved in.

Change up your foods on a regular basis.

When you're using intermittent fasting, you want to rotate your foods and calories according to your schedule. On the days that you're working out, you'll want to eat a little bit more. On the days that you're resting, you'll want to reduce the calories that you're consuming. This will help balance out the calories so that you're building muscles when you're working out and burning fat while you're not working out. Cutting down a little on rest days should be easy since you won't need the extra calories. It will be a mental workout instead of a physical one. During those rest days, you'll be going through more of your fat stores than otherwise.

However, besides the calorie counts, you need to make sure that you're also looking at the nutrients that you're eating. More protein on days that you're working out will help you a lot. When you're taking it easy, you'll need a slightly different nutrient set. If you keep changing up your carbs and protein by when you're working out and resting, then you'll find yourself becoming a leaner, fit person quite quickly.

There are no shortcuts when it comes to dieting and fasting.

When people hear stories about losing tons of weight in a short amount of time, they get excited about the diet. When they try it, and it doesn't work in a week, they feel disappointed and often give up. The short term view of dieting and fasting gets in the way of actually losing weight. Instead of thinking about the seven days in a week individually, you would do better to focus on the longer term and think about what you're eating over the course of a week. Instead of micromanaging your hours, focus on the day as a whole and getting the nutrients in at some point during the day.

Your body won't care about when the nutrients get into your body. Whether it's a protein shake one hour or twelve hours later, your body will still get the protein. You just need to ensure that you are getting the calories and nutrients necessary for your health and fitness. You're just shifting when exactly those get to your body in an intermittent fasting schedule. If you focus on the longer term, you'll realize that ultimately fasting will do you good.

When fasting, you will want less food.

On a fast, you slowly pull away from the restraints of your food addictions and diet. You'll be eating because you want to, not because you are on a schedule that dictates when you will eat. This change

won't be obvious at first. It may take weeks or months or maybe even a year before you're free from those cravings that you used to have. As time passes, you'll feel more comfortable fasting. You won't crave food as you did before. You may even develop a better appreciation for food when you do eat. Your mind will think of eating as something other than the chore that it is when you're not on an intermittent fast. It will be an extremely enjoyable time, instead of just something that you have to do.

Losing fat and building muscle doesn't happen at the same time.

If you're looking to not only lose fat but also gain muscle, then you'll have to do some specific things with your intermittent fasting to get it to work with you. You'll have to use calorie cycling as well to help you get to the gains and losses that you want in your body. To lose weight, you'll need to be taking in fewer calories than you're burning off. But for muscle gain, you'll need to have enough calories and nutrients to help your muscles along. So the two processes are already at odds because you can't have a calorie deficit for weight loss and a calorie surplus for muscle gain at the same time.

If you consider longer time frames, you might begin to see how the two working together can make you a better you.

You will get a better result if you train a little less while fasting.

When you're fasting, you should consider a long-term when you look at your training. Instead of daily goals, pick out goals for the week's workout sessions. Once you've decided that, make sure that you're doing the most important and effective exercises first. Doing compound exercises early will help you get the most out of your fast. You may decide on the way to split the workout through the day. You could use the upper body in the morning and lower body in the afternoon. It could look more like pushups in the morning and squats in the afternoon.

Your workouts will be much more effective during a fast because of the changes going on in your body. Both hormonal and metabolic changes are happening. These changes will mean that you'll need less training to get the same amount of change. Intermittent fasting will allow your body to change more quickly and more efficiently. Less time will mean that you've got more time to pursue other goals. It's a win for you in every way.

Drinking a lot of water will help you throughout fasting.

One of the most important things to remember while using intermittent fasting is that you need to keep yourself hydrated. Your needs may be different than someone else, but the general rule is to drink around two liters of water every day. You may not feel like you want to or need it, but you should do it anyways. Your body will only tell you that it's thirty when it is dehydrated. This is something to be avoided.

Humans obtain some of our water from the foods we consume. There are some foods, like vegetables, which are more efficient at providing water content. Because you will be eating less, you won't be getting an extra water boost throughout the day. Drinking water often will help counter the loss.

Water may also help you battle hunger pains during the day. It'll help you conquer the mental battle not to eat all the time. There aren't many problems that can come from drinking water, so you should consume lots of it to help with the intermittent fast that you're on. Other liquids are allowed, but water will be the most beneficial to them all.

The best diet is the one that works for your body.

Everyone wants the easy road to the best possible life. They want it to be something that will dramatically change them quick. Diet books sell like crazy because people are always looking for that one thing that will improve their lives so much. A quick fix is what they're looking for. However, the quick fix rarely works. Everyone is slightly different, and

diets will affect them differently. Not all diets will take into account every single thing, like gender, age, body type, fitness levels, medical conditions, or allergies. All of these things, and more contribute to how your body works. You won't be able to follow a quick fix probably because of these reasons. To find what works for your body, you're going to need some time and patience to experiment and see what works best.

Intermittent fasting does well in this regard. While using this method for weight loss, you can experiment with how your eating schedule and patterns are set up. This experimentation won't cause harm to your body and health. As you experiment, there will be foods and eating schedules that make you feel full of energy and ones that make you feel lethargic or otherwise unhealthy. As you figure out what is and isn't working, you'll be slowly tweaking your life to make it into a better one. This is one of the reasons why intermittent fasting is so much better than most other diets. You're not restricted to the foods you eat, just the amount of time that you have to eat.

Eat-Stop-Eat

Once or twice each week, you will fast for twenty-four hours. As an illustration, you would eat dinner one morning and not eat again until the following morning. Most professionals say if you make it to twenty hours; it is okay.
To further condition your body, for two days eat about 2,500 calories if you are a man and 2,000 if you are a woman. After several regular eating days, attempt another fasting, and repeat the agenda.

Non-Fasting and Fasting Day Nutrients

For the days on an active fast, try not consume many calories. You can drink sparkling or plain water, diet soda, coffee, or tea. When the fast is complete, eat what you like using restraint. Enjoy plenty of veggies, fruits, and take advantage of the spices for variety.

Protein should be apparent using twenty to thirty grams of high-quality protein. Consume a total of one-hundred grams every four to five hours. You can use protein powders if needed. If you are gaining extra pounds during in between your fasting schedule, consider cutting back by approximately 10% on the amount of food you consume on non-fasting days.

Some individuals cannot 'hack' the plan and state it makes him/her less adaptable to enjoying time with friends at social gatherings. Many have issues of crankiness and headaches which can lead to the plan's failure.

With that said, the plan's benefits are overwhelming because you can judge your progress, and you choose to eat. It takes learning some self-control, but you can get it.

Note: Never fast two consecutive days. Also, you should not take the challenge more than two fasting days in one week.

Fluid Intake

With a strict plan such as this one, you must remain hydrated. You can drink plenty of clear liquids but where are the nutrients. On your fasting days, stick to apple juice water, broth, cranberry juice, ice pops, plain gelatin, black coffee or tea. This is okay since you will be fasting for twenty to twenty-four hours.

You can also enjoy foods including ice cream, skim milk, juice with pulp, or strained creamy soup. Try a whey protein supplemental shake or some low-fat frozen yogurt. These choices will provide some essential nutrients, fiber, as well as the necessary calorie counts. Just be sure to use low-calorie juices, ice cream, and a few ice cubes for a smoothie treat.

It is advisable to confer with your physician before you begin this or any other dieting plan. While you are fasting, you might need to discontinue any dietary supplements or medications. According to research at Vanderbilt University, daily liquid diets will provide you between 400 to 800 calories.

Additional Tips

With this fasting method, it is essential not to fall into a habit of fasting and binging because it will create havoc within your body. It is more than your body can handle since the cycle will only work for individuals who can practice control and moderate consumption of food. It is recommended by the professionals to perform resistance-style weight training on the days you aren't fasting.

Try a minimal yoga session or light cardio exercise if you are complete 'out of it' on your fasting days. Any more vigorous exercising could make it difficult to achieve the time allotment of your fasting schedule. Remember, at first—it is common to feel angered, anxious, fatigued, or have headaches. This will pass once your body adjusts to the new dieting plan.

Try to keep in mind; every single day you can successfully stay on your desired plan; is one more day toward your successful 30-day goal.

Understanding Your Body

Insulin Resistance

The modern way of life has made us to neglect tasting forcing our bodies to spend more time in the feeding window. This forces the body cells to mobilize and burn less fat for energy whereas the pathway for burning glucose gets overused. Eventually, the level of insulin in the body remains high forcing the body to rely on glucose and avoid burning fat. This chronic exposure is harmful to our bodies because it can lead to insulin resistance which results in secretion of excess insulin when your body is in feeding window. Some of the common metabolic syndrome (abdominal fat storage, obesity, high triglycerides, elevated glucose, and low HDL) occurs a result of chronic insulin resistance. If you grow to be insulin resistant your body will predominately burn fat and rare ever get the chance to burn fat. And when you run out of glucose your body never transit to the fasted state but you get hungry.

Fat Adaptation

Your body has the ability to become 'fat-adapted' rely on stored fat for energy rather than glucose. However, if it is not used to it, it will take your precious time and practice. You will have to do something to upgrade all your fat burning pathways. These includes increasing insulin sensitivity in a bid to lower insulin and promoting mobilization of fat into free fatty acids right from the adipocytes. Some of the best way of improving your fat adaptation include;

- Intermittent fasting: when you widen the fasting window you increase the ability of your body to burn more fat.

- Eating low carb high-fat diet: this signals the body to burn/mobilize fat for energy instead of using glucose since you avail less glucose and more fat all the time.

- Caloric restriction: as discussed earlier caloric restriction has all the benefits of IF. During caloric restriction, less glucose is availed for fuel forcing your body to rely heavily on stored fat for energy.

- Exercise: glucose is high depleted during high-intensity exercise, glycogen is not spare either. Your body is then forced to switch over and mobilize n more stored fat for energy. This ends up improving your insulin sensitivity.

Metabolic Exercise

Intermittent fasting is the best strategy to strengthen your body's ability to persist in the fasted state. It is the best exercise you can give to your body to help it burn fat instead of continually mobilizing glucose for energy.

Like any other exercise, it will take time before your body achieves this, compare it to building muscles. Also, just like in muscle atrophy this ability degrades once you stop exercising. Widening the fasting window is actually the most appropriate way of achieving the best results. Physical exercise can be compared to fasting in terms of the benefits it brings. This what physical exercise can do ;

- Decrease insulin level.
- Decrease blood glucose
- Increase sensitivity to insulin
- Increase mobilization of free fatty acids and lipolysis.
- Increase oxidation of cellular fat
- Increase glucagon
- Increase growth hormone.

All the above can be accomplished by doing nothing, no exercise! The secret is widening the fasting window only, and you will achieve all these benefits. When you extend the time, your body spends in the fasted state you subject it to a form of metabolic "exercise." You are training the body to efficiently and rapidly mobilize stored body fat for energy. Things will get better and better as you continue fasting thereby lengthening your metabolic practice.

More Fasting, Less Feeding

How do you achieve long-lasting and effortless fat loss? Many people are always in a dilemma when it comes to losing fat. But it's simple, train your body to survive on 2 meals a day. Leveraging your overnight fast is the easiest way of accomplishing fat loss. The rule is simple, skip

breakfast, take lighter lunch, and end the day with larger dinner. By

doing, so your body will learn to automatically shift between parasympathetic (rest and digest) and sympathetic (flight) nervous system tone. This is because activation and alertness from the sympathetic tone will be increased by under eating during the day while the parasympathetic tone will be higher during the fed state.

When in the fasted state your body will burn fat that is inaccessible during fed state. And since it enters the fasted state after roughly 12 hours, if you do not skip the first meal of the day you will rarely enter the fasted state. This is the major reason why when you are starting fasting you lose fat quickly without making any other change to your diet.

Avoid Carbohydrates

Refined carbohydrates should be avoided because they overdrive the feeding window since they raise insulin and glucose levels more than other macronutrients. When you take a meal, it will take your body a few hours to work on the food you have consumed, then burn as much as it can from these foods.

When you take refined carbohydrates, your body will easily burn energy since its readily available, neglecting the stored fats.

Exercise Is Important

Your body can easily get fat-adapted via exercises. The body depletes glycogen (stored glucose) during fasting, it's further depleted during training. When glycogen is depleted insulin sensitivity is improved. When you take a meal immediately after workouts, the body can store it efficiently as glycogen or burn it for energy to aid the recovery process. This leads to less fat being stored.

How Intermittent Fasting Affects Your Metabolism

Most people have the idea that skipping meals leads to a slow metabolic rate because your body will need to preserve as much energy as it can. Well, it is true that extremely long periods without food can lead to a slower metabolism, but studies have also shown that fasting for short periods increases your metabolism and not slow it down. One study published in NCBI conducted on 11 healthy men proved that a 3 day fast increased their metabolism by a notable 14%!

This was thought to be because of the rise of the hormone known as norepinephrine, which promotes the burning of fat. This hormone is a stress hormone that improves attention and alertness and has some other effects on the body. One of them is instructing the body's fat cells to release fatty acids. The more the norepinephrine is in your bloodstream, the larger the amounts of fatty acids that are availed for your body to burn.

Other ways that intermittent fasting impacts your metabolism positively include the following:

1: Eliminating wastes

It is normal for toxins to accumulate in your system during ordinary drinking and eating. During intermittent fasting, your body can eliminate those toxins and wastes (as you get to regularly clear your digestive system) hence cleansing your internal organs. This, in turn, increases your metabolism as there are no toxins to hinder digestion.

As you cut down on particular foods at particular times during intermittent fasting, your system gets a window where it can cleanse itself and remove toxins and wastes. So when you get to eat, your body doesn't have to use energy for both digestion and removing toxins- it can fully focus on digestion and other processes in the system.

Intermittent fasting also regulates digestion. Slow digestion negatively affects your body's ability to break down food and burn fat. A clear bowel is a healthy bowel, and on a fast, your body has less to digest thus reducing the work that the system has to carry out. This promotes healthy bowel and metabolic function.

2: Trains the body to burn fat

When you are fasting, your body is temporarily deprived of the normal sugars that it is usually used to burning for fuel- the sugars would be used as the primary source of fuel. This forces your body to turn on the fat burning metabolism to meet its energy requirements.

This ensures you burn fat in the short term (during your fast) and also resets your body to depend more on fat for energy during normal eating (as the body will be expecting less food). This means that your metabolism will improve from glucose burning to fat burning.

3: Regulates blood sugar

Most people associate eating with gnawing feelings of deep hunger. But the thing is; hunger is majorly caused by shifts in blood sugar levels. With intermittent fasting, your body burns fat (and not sugars) at a steady rate hence keeping your hunger under control since there is no frequent conversion and stagnation of blood sugars in the system. Also, as your body burns fat for energy, this leaves behind a satiating feeling, which you cannot experience if you are in the fed state where blood glucose levels are high.

This means that the level of insulin in the system is also reduced, a phenomenon that lowers the risk of insulin resistance (where insulin becomes ineffective) making sure that digestion and metabolism in general, stays perfect.

4: Better eating habits

Fasting also certainly changes your attitude towards food in that you become less dependent on it and in turn gain more clarity about what you will be eating and what's best for you. Once you know what's necessary for your body to optimum function, you will be led to eating right, which will energize your metabolism. For instance, eating right could mean that you incorporate more fiber, which leads to easier digestion of foods.

5: Slowing down of the aging process

When you give your body a rest from normal digestion through fasting, your body can be able to slow down aging, as it has less overall work to perform. This gives your digestive system a break, as you will be eating less. This can boost your metabolism so that more fat is burned down, which leads to inevitable weight loss.
This is significant because one of the major consequences of aging is a slower metabolism. The younger your body stays, the more efficient and faster your metabolism will be.

Role in Fat Loss and Building Muscle

Two important outcomes, which result in effective fat loss and muscle gain, happen when you go on intermittent fasting:

Your insulin sensitivity is improved. Whenever you eat, your body produces insulin to help it absorb the nutrients from the foods you ate.

Insulin carries glucose from your blood stream to your muscles, liver and fat cells, which stores excess glucose for use later when energy levels are low. After the insulin transports the glucose from your bloodstream to your muscles, liver, and fat cells, the latter will later on utilize your blood sugar for energy. When fat cells store too much glucose their sensitivity to insulin weakens which not only increases your risk of cancer and heart disease, but also hinders your ability to shed off fat from your body.

To help you address the issue with insulin sensitivity, you eat less frequently (which is what intermittent fasting lets you accomplish, especially when done on a regular basis) so that your body ends up producing insulin with less frequency. This results in your body having a heightened sensitivity to insulin, which leads to easier fat loss, muscle gain, and improved overall health.

Your body's growth hormone is increased. Growth hormone, or GH, is the reason why subjecting your body to intermittent fasting lets you lose fat as well as gain muscle. This hormone supports your body as it builds new muscular tissue and burn off fat; it also helps strengthen your bones, improve your physical function, and give your longevity a boost.

You can increase your GH levels by going on intermittent fasts, especially if you complement these with adequate sleep and regular weight training. Because the effect of your increased GH levels only lasts as long as your fast, it is important that you do intermittent fasting on a regular basis to achieve your desired results (losing fat and building muscles).

Foods and Drinks Allowed

When you choose to do intermittent fasting, you do not have anything besides water. You can have a cup of plain tea or coffee in the morning, but you can do away with sugarless gums or diet drinks.

Number of Calories to be consumed

Although intermittent fasting is requires being strict about which foods to fuel your body with and which to avoid, it does not require you to obsess over measuring every meal precisely. Yes, you do have to keep track of the calories you consume and the calories you burn but you can be fairly flexible with it. It helps to think about losing fat and building muscle through intermittent fasting as a long-term goal, and not as a daily battle. What's important is that you focus on eating real foods and on keeping your calorie intake at a healthy low (as opposed to severely restricting it to the point of your body suffering from nutrient deficiencies) most of the time.

Calories Needed For Fat Loss

Caloric requirements depend if it is a weight training day or an off/cardio only day. To determine calories required for fat loss, you must first identify the calories needed for maintenance. The easiest way to get an estimate is to multiply your weight in pounds by 15. For example, if you weigh 200 lbs, the total calories needed for maintenance would be 3000 calories per day.

Calorie requirements for weight training days

To determine calories on weight training days, take some maintenance calories and add 500 to it. So, for our 200 lb person, they would be eating 3500 calories on days that they lift.

Calorie requirements for off or cardio days

To determine calories needed for off or cardio days, just divide your maintenance calories in half. So, for off or cardio days, our 200 lb person would be eating 1500 calories per day.

Macronutrient Breakdown

Now that your calorie requirements for fat loss have been determined, it's time to figure out how much of each macronutrient you will be needing. The amounts will vary on if you are weight training that day or not. The macronutrients we will be using will be the big three:

- Fat
- Protein
- Carbohydrates

(Be sure to remember that fat has 9 calories per gram and protein and carbs each have 4 calories per gram.)

Macronutrient breakdown for weight training days

- Fat

The maximum amount of fat eaten per day is 30 Grams. It doesn't matter where the fat comes from, as long as 10 of these grams are in the form of Omega-3 Fish Oil.

- Protein

To determine the minimum amount of protein per day, you multiply your weight by 1.25. Our 200 lb person will need a minimum of 250g of protein to preserve muscle. Sources don't matter, just be sure to be mindful that you don't exceed the fat limit. Chicken, very lean red meat, fat-free cheese and protein powder (whey or casein) are excellent choices.

- Carbohydrates

Carbohydrates make up the remaining calories in your diet. Once again, sources don't matter, just be sure not to exceed the 30g fat limit and be you want to keep sugar below 100 grams. So, in our sample person, he is getting 270 calories from fat and 1000 calories from protein. With the caloric goal on lifting days being 3500, that leaves him with 2230 calories left for carbs. Divide 2230 by 4, and you come up with a maximum carbohydrate amount of ~558 grams.

Macronutrient breakdown for non-lifting or cardio days

As mentioned earlier, calories needed for days that you don't weight train or do cardio are 1/2 of what your maintenance calories are. Here is the macronutrient breakdown:

- Fat

Again, the amount of fat is unchanged from training days. The maximum amount of fat eaten per day is 30 Grams. It doesn't matter where the fat comes from, as long as 10 of these grams are in the form of Omega-3 Fish Oil.

- Carbohydrates

On rest day's or cardio only days, carbohydrate sources should only come from fibrous green vegetables and the trace amounts found in your protein sources, such as whey and cheese. The maximum amount per day should not exceed 20 grams.

- Protein

The minimum amount of protein is your weight in pounds x 1.25. For our sample person requiring 1500 calories per day, he would be getting 270 calories from fat, 80 calories from carbohydrates and the remaining 1150 calories from protein. That would equal to ~287.5 grams.

Diet for Weight Training Days

Weight training will be a 3 day a week, full body routine. You can use Monday-Wednesday-Friday, but the days are up to you, as long as there is a day off between workouts.

Pre-Workout
- On training days, the fast is broken with a whey protein/carb shake, 15-30 minutes before your workout begins.
- A mix of simple carbs and whey protein is recommended.
- Protein =.25g/lb x weight Carbs =.25g/lb x weight
- Gatorade powder (not the pre-made liquid form) or a maltodextrin/dextrose blend is my pre-workout carb of choice. Keep fat to a minimum here.

Post-Workout
- Within 30 minutes of your workout, you have another shake, but this time, use a whey + casein/dextrose mix.
- Protein =.25g/lb x weight Carbs =.50g/lb x weight

The Rest of the day

Your first solid food meal of the day is 1 hour after your PWO shake. It will be the biggest meal of the day. Remaining meal times are up to you, but you should be tapering your calories down until your last meal. Remember that with Intermittent Fasting you don't need to eat every 2-3 hours. Just make sure that you meet your caloric/macronutrient goals. It is recommended that you make a casein shake right before the eating period is over. Since it's a slow digesting protein, it will help keep you full longer.

Diet for Off or Cardio Days

Since calories are significantly reduced on off or cardio days, the eating window is shorter. It works best to have 2-3 good size meals, rather than the 6-7 you read about in muscle mags.

On cardio days, the fast is broken with a 50g protein shake, 1 hour after cardio is complete. Two hours after the shake, have your first "real" meal and continue until the 6 hours are up. As mentioned earlier, carbs are limited to 20 per day and should consist of fibrous green vegetables and the trace amounts of food.

Intermittent Fasting Diet Weight Training Routine
Weight training is a full body 3-day routine. Again, specific days don't matter but make sure you have a day off in between workouts. You will be working the large muscles only (legs, back, chest) on days 1 and 2 and will add in the smaller muscles arms/calves) on day 3. You will do 4 sets of 6-8 reps for each large muscle and 2-3 sets of 8-12 for the smaller ones.

Here is a sample workout routine:
- Day 1: Push
- Flat Bench Press / Shoulder Press / Leg Press / Weighted Crunches

- Day 2: Pull
- Rows / Chinups / Hamstring Curl

- Day 3: Push/Pull
Incline Bench Press / Rows / Squats / Calf Raises / Lateral Raise / Barbell Curl / Tricep Pushdown / Lateral Raise / Back Extensions / Weighted Crunches

For maximum fat loss, cardio should be down 2-3 times per week. Start with a 5-minute warm up and then begin 10 minutes of High-Intensity Interval Training, or HIIT. It works best on an elliptical or a spin bike, instead of a treadmill. You will do this in 1-minute intervals. Max intensity for 1 minute, followed by a moderate pace for 1 minute. Repeat until 10 minutes are up.

After, the HIIT session is over, drink some water and rest for 5 minutes. After, your rest, do 30 minutes of Low to Moderate Intensity, Steady State Cardio. A treadmill works great for this. Don't forget to wait an hour and have your 50g of protein.

Comparing Intermittent Fasting With Diet Fads

A lot of people are talking about intermittent fasting, but still, there are many who are questioning "what is it?" Often known as short-term fasting, it is one of the best method used in weight loss programs. People experiencing intermittent fasting have proved that it does not cause starvation, tiredness, and other symptoms of the daily diet. It is because it is not the same with diet fad. It is entirely different with completely different results.

Everyone already knows diet as a general way of losing fat. It is free of charge, straightforward and easy. However, the effect it gives is, not even if compared to the hard work someone must go through in dieting. Surely diet will help in losing weight, but it will not be a drastic change, and this change will probably take place after a few weeks of dieting. It is where the difference lies between diet and intermittent fasting. Following a flexible short-term fasting will give an incredible result.

Not only will it reduce weight fast but also show a drastic change in the body. This method affects the lifestyle of those doing the weight loss program. So, it can be a long-lasting weight loss program. Another difference is the phrase 'burn fat feed muscle' applies in intermittent fasting. Many people have proved while following this type of method they did not lose any muscle mass.

Knowing the differences leads to a conclusion. Based on the facts given, short-term fasting is one step ahead in succeeding to weight loss compared to diet fad. Succeeding in the results and also the process. It is a lifetime program which is far from regrettable.

Lose Weight - Diets Don't Work, Intermittent Fasting Does

To lose weight, you need to burn more calories than you are taking in on a consistent basis. Nothing too profound there. The problem that most people have when attempting to lose weight is that they make it more difficult that it needs to be. If you keep it simple and stick with it, you will achieve the results that you are looking for.

If your diet depends on you counting every calorie, weighing your food, and restricting your intake to the point that you are miserable, you will ▢uit before any noticeable results are achieved. For a diet to get results, it needs to restrict your calories in a way that is easy to follow and allows you to maintain some sense of normalcy in your life. Most of them don't do this, which is why diets don't work, at least not in the long term.

Intermittent fasting is the best way to lose weight. Before you get too worried about fasting and think that you can't do it, here's explanation. Intermittent fasting allows you to eat every day still as well as eat the same way that you normally do. It is far less restrictive than other diet plans and is the best long-term solution. If you fast twice a week, you will decrease your caloric intake by 20 percent per week. It will cause you to lose significant weight as well as let you still eat the foods that you love.

If you typically eat 2,500 calories a day and fast twice per week, you should cut your calories by around 3,500 per week.
*   2500 X 7 days = 17,500
*   17,500 X 20% = 3,500

3,500 calories make up a pound of fat which will equate to losing around a pound of fat a week. Intermittent fasting is a long-term solution and can be used for as long as you like. If you need to lose a little amount of fat, it can help you to get lean and have your six-pack showing all summer long. If you need to lose a lot of fat, you can use fasting as long as it takes to reach your goal.

If you think that a pound a week isn't enough, think again. Any of these claims that people can lose 15 pounds in a week are usually bogus, are mostly water weight, and are not long term.

If they worked so well, people wouldn't need to try ten different diets a year and yo-yo their weight up and down every time. It's time for you to quit searching for the next fad diet and put your weight loss problems behind you. Give intermittent fasting a try and watch the fat melt off week by week.

Tips to Successful Intermittent Fasting

If you are planning to start fasting intermittently here are some key pointer to consider.

Don't Try When At The First Week Of Your Ketogenic/Low-Carb Diet

It's important to note that intermittent fasting should not be tried during the first weeks of ketogenic/low-carb diet or when following a standard American diet. Your body should first adapt to ketogenic diet prior to trying any IF protocol. When you get used to ketogenic diet, your body will learn to utilize ketones instead of glucose for energy. Any attempt to start IF straight way will not succeed. Instead, your body will become glucose-dependent, and this will make you too hungry to follow any IF protocol. Remember intermittent fasting is a gradual process which should be natural not to make you feel hungry or struggle.

Listen To Your Body

When done naturally intermittent fasting delivers fantastic results. Try to be as natural as possible when following your IF protocol. For example, when it's time for lunch, and you are not hungry, you do not have to eat, skip it. If it's too late to take your dinner, skip it and have a larger breakfast.

However, IF requires a lot of restrictions and control especially during the fasting window. If you are prone to unhealthy eating habits, it can be one of the triggers to overindulgence to unhealthy behaviors. Therefore, you should be very careful when trying any of the IF protocols.

Don't Force Yourself

Never deprive or restrict yourself in the name of intermittent fasting, it should be as natural as possible. First train your body to become fat adapted and the hunger sessions will be minimal. The best way to achieving this is starting slow, avoid taking snacks between your meals and as you get used to it tart skipping one of the regular meals, preferably breakfast.

IF is a lifestyle change and to succeed you need to ease your way in. Give it a trial run and see if it's something you can comfortably adopt. Try a single plan, for example, try a 24-hour fast or maybe follow partial fasting that will include an eight-hour eating window. If the trial plan works and the experience is tolerable, you can now work with an ongoing plan.

Eat Well When The Feeding Window Opens

Eating well means eating healthy. One of the biggest challenges of intermittent fasting is over-consuming during the feeding window. You do not have to restrict your food intake, but it's also healthy to prioritize taking whole foods.

To enjoy the benefits of intermittent fasting, you should never counteract the calorie deficit created during the fasting periods. For this reason, you should avoid overzealous bingeing on processed sugars/carbs.

Keep Yourself Busy

A busy schedule will help you to skip meals naturally. Also, avoid spending much of your time near your kitchen because this can tempt you to take a treat even when not feeling hungry. If you immerse yourself in a serious activity, your attention will be diverted from cravings and put into good use. This can be of great importance than you ever imagined, just don't let yourself to fall into boredom. Stay engaged and take part in the most energy-intensive tasks.

Understand If Doenst Fix Everything

IF has the potential to help you live longer and lose weight but you should fully understand that this is just but one of the methods to help your realize your targets. You should consider other factors like sufficient sleep, stress levels, exercise, micronutrients & macronutrients when striving to achieve your targets. IF should never be used as a quick fix for consumption of more than required carbs. It should be done naturally with feeling deprived or restricted.

Create Leverage

The list of the benefits you get from IF is endless. But, you should remember that the magnitude of these benefits during the first few days or weeks will hugely depend on your will power. Human beings are hardwired, and the probability of taking action to avoid pain is 10 times higher than taking action to gain pleasure.

Challenge yourself and play with your mind using 'negative' goals. Just imagine something awful will happen if you fail to fast more often. Creating a leverage will put every part of your body in the mood to fast more naturally.

IF Is Not For Everone

This is a warning, intermittent fasting is not for you if you suffer from type 1 diabetes, bulimia nervosa, or anorexia nervosa.
However, type 2 diabetics can do intermittent fasting only under the guidance of a doctor. This is because such people require medical

adjustments to succeed in their IF and at the same time benefit from the medication.

Studies have shown that breastfeeding and pregnant women should also avoid intermittent fasting. IF is not effective as a weight loss tool for women especially the pre-menopausal women.

What To Eat

Sure, the term "intermittent fasting" or "fasting" means not eating. However, this diet is not about starving yourself. It is also not about obsessively counting each calorie present in your food and drinks. This is not a CRaP (calorie restriction as primary) type of diet. IF firmly believes that starving yourself is setting yourself up for failure. You won't get healthy if you starve yourself. You won't beef up if you do not feed your muscles. You will not experience steady weight loss if you starve yourself.

Intermittent fasting is giving your body the right amount of calories it needs to perform its many functions. Then why does it include fasting? What will fasting aim to achieve?

Imagine your body as a paper shredder. Eating is like feeding the shredder with a bunch of papers. Fasting is similar to pausing from inserting (feeding) paper to the shredder. This pause allows the machine to process what you just fed it.

 Try cramming batches of a paper nonstop to the paper shredder. Soon, you will have problems such as jamming.
This same thing happens in the body. If you keep feeding, it will put its efforts into digesting and storing food with the intention of dealing with it later. The body has the natural inclination to work on food it has at hand, store it for later burning when all the food has been digested. If you keep on eating, the body can't convert and use energy.

Research has demonstrated that eating small meals frequently is not going to help you with weight loss. It won't have a lasting positive effect on your metabolism either. Constant eating is not going to give your body time to process food completely. It will constantly trigger the system to break down foods with little time for doing anything else. You have to let your body rest from processing foods and let it turn its attention to other important things like burning fat and building muscles.

Research has also demonstrated that eating large and infrequent meals is better than eating smaller and more frequent meals. Larger and less frequent meals increase satiety, especially if these are high in proteins. This type of meals will help you feel fuller longer. This is especially helpful if you are going on a fast in a few hours after eating.

On a fast, you do not eat anything. That is ideal. For some, 16 hours of 0 calories may be quite a challenge. Intermittent fasting is not that strict. It does not require absolute zero intakes during the fasting periods. You may eat during the fast periods, but not as much as in regular eating. Remember, you may eat, but in limited amounts and from within a narrowed list of foods.

Water

This is a must when you are in a fast. You have to drink water. Drinking large amounts of water for many reasons is critical. First, during a fast, you will stimulate several cellular processes that will produce wastes and by-products. It is crucial to eliminate these soon to prevent accumulation within the tissues, which can result in unpleasant symptoms.

Drinking water during a fast helps curb hunger and fight cravings. Most often, when we feel hungry, we are thirsty. This is a helpful trick to stave off hunger. When you drink water, your stomach expands - much like when you eat food. The expansion of the stomach muscles will trigger certain stretch receptors that will send a message to the brain. The message will tell the brain to stop feeling or thinking of hunger. Nice trick, huh?

Another good trick is to add certain calorie-free herbs and spices in water with natural appetite-suppressive effects. Add a pinch of cinnamon to your drinking water to combat hunger and cravings. You may also infuse lemon slices to water to suppress hunger and cravings further. Not just that, these add-ons can help in detoxifying your body, taking your fast further.

Tea or Coffee (black)

This is the wildcard for the fast periods. Some IF practitioners take a cup of coffee or tea in the morning to help them extend their fast until their first meal of the day around lunchtime.

A few studies on coffee found that a cup in the morning can increase your body's fat burning potential. Black coffee has been demonstrated to help in curbing hunger in the morning. On the IF, black coffee can boost the fat burning process.

When taking tea or coffee, black is the way to go. You get the full
goodness of various active compounds. Adding sugar and/or cream will
provide calories in the body that can break your fast.
Green tea is also an acceptable drink in the morning to help you get
through. It also has a lot of health benefits, including increased
metabolism, better energy, and even cancer prevention.

Gum (?)
No. some people on a fast report that chewing sugar-free gum helped
them through the 16-hour fast. However, this is not recommended.
Some artificial sweeteners in gum can be converted into sugar by the
digestive system. These sugars can turn into calories and break your
fast. In addition, some gum ingredients may be bad for health and upset
the balance of healthy gut bacteria.

Foods to eat in between fasts

This is also known as "what to eat during the window period." This is one
of the best points in the 8:16 intermittent fasting diet. You can eat
whatever you want. Yes, it does not require complicated food lists or
fancy food preparations.

However, if you want to get amazing results in the soonest possible
time, you have to be smart about food choices in between fasts.
One problem with most of the foods we eat is that they contain too
many calories with little nutritional value. Foods made of highly
processed ingredients like refined flour, refined sugar and high fructose
corn syrup (HCFS) make up most of our diets.

These kinds of foods make it difficult to achieve energy balance in the
body. Eat more veggies and meats, instead. These are low in calories
but very filling. Vegetables, for instance, are great at making you feel
full longer, but they have low-calorie content. If you eat 2 cups of
vegetables, you will be eating a lot and will feel full for hours. The
calories are still low even with the larger servings.

Continuing The Plan

The secret to success in fasting is consistency. As we have emphasized,
find a method that suits your body and stick to it. Make sure you
integrate it into your daily schedule thereby making it a habit on busy
days or weekends. Here are some tips to help you during the weekends
and while eating outside your home.

Tips for the weekend

- Hit the gym and do some light body stretching exercises
- Catch up on your reading
- Make sure you sleep early.
- Go for a walk or do errands
- Meet your friends. Don't stay at home doing nothing or watching the television
- Avoid the clock. Looking at it will not prepare your mind for the fast
- Eat a lot of vegetables and lean proteins during the weekend
- Go for a movie in the cinemas

Tips for outdoor eating

One of the things you should put in place while fasting is your kitchen. The pre-fasting meal and the post-fasting meal have to be planned to suit your purpose for the fast. It is always advisable to prepare your meals so as to monitor what you eat.

It is understandable that some occasions may arise that will require an outdoor eating. It may be a friend's birthday party, wedding, lunch invitations, etc. the bottom line is to do what suits your program. All you need to do is to drink water and continue with your fast.

We said earlier that you don't need to advertise your fasting to avoid negative opinion. So when you are in situations like this, try and tactically avoid being forced to eat so as to maintain your schedule.

Exercise and Intermittent Fasting

One common question people have when doing intermittent fasting is whether or not it is safe and healthy to exercise either aerobically or anaerobically while they are, say, "running on empty." Freak out the Jackson Browne! But, if done correctly, the combination can help you burn lots of your body's fat reserves quickly. Maintaining some exercise routine is vital for your mental and physical health – that's a given. So, in fact, exercising and running in a fasted state is a great way to become fat adapted and improve your mental state at the same time.

You've already heard the adage, 80% diet, 20% exercise – to combine dieting with exercise. This is true! Imagine if we could make our body burn more fat for fuel while at rest, and then also burn fat more efficiently during exercise. Most of us have 40,000 calories of fat in our bodies at any given time and around 1,200 calories of muscle glycogen or sugar. Imagine how far or how much we could exercise if we had access to that 40,000-calorie fuel tank. That's 33 times the amount of energy fuel! So, perhaps next time you run out of energy in the middle of an exercise routine, you will wish your body was in fat-burning mode instead of calorie-burning mode.

The first step to burning more fat during exercise is: you need to have what's called an "aerobic base." The way to build this base is through aerobic heart rate training, which will raise what is known as your "aerobic capacity." Aerobic capacity is defined as the maximal amount of oxygen in milliliters (ml) that an athlete utilizes in one minute, per kilogram of body weight. In layman's terms, the higher the "aerobic base" or "capacity," the more body work you can do in one minute. The best method I have found for heart rate training is Phil Maffetone's "MAF" training.

What does this mean for exercise? Technically, by having a higher aerobic base, we boost the size and strength of our heart, the concentration of hemoglobin in our blood, the density of our capillaries, and the number of mitochondria in our muscles. The benefits expand beyond the scope of this book, but essentially by developing an aerobic base, we become healthier inside and out.

What this means for intermittent fasting is that when you are training in a fasted state, your body becomes superbly efficient at burning fat for fuel. From an aerobic aspect your body can more efficiently utilize oxygen and this, in turn, makes you more efficient at exercise aerobically or anaerobically. You must first develop your aerobic base to enhance anaerobic exercise.

If you are looking to add muscle, fasting can help by increasing the production of certain hormones in your body. Other than weight training and getting the proper amount of sleep regularly, fasting has proven to be one of the most effective methods of increasing human growth hormone, or "HGH." Studies have also suggested that fasting in combination with regular exercise can increase the levels of testosterone in men and women, which is another hormone that can decrease body fat and increase muscle mass. Here are my recommendations for adding muscle:

• Don't push yourself too hard. If you are doing "cardio" exercise, as a test, make sure you can carry on a conversation at the same time; otherwise, you may be pushing yourself too hard. When you are doing the exercise slowly, but for a long time, that's when your body is becoming more "fat adapted." That's when it is going into a ketogenic state. Listen always to your body, and stop if you start to feel dizzy or lightheaded.

• The 16/8 method, in particular, recommends scheduling your meals for when you plan to finish doing any moderate-to-intense exercise. Plan your high-intensity workouts for around a time when you are getting ready to break your fast so that you can eat soon after that. Properly scheduled, if your workout is very intense, you can follow it with a carbohydrate-rich snack.

•   If you are lifting weights, make sure you are getting adequate protein or supplementing with adequate BCAAs. "Feast" on meals that are high in protein. Eating protein on a regular basis is vital to muscle growth.

•   When planning your meals with workouts in mind, try combining fast-acting simple carbohydrates with a protein that will serve to stabilize your blood sugar after your workout. A banana and some peanut butter is a good example.

Here are some sample routines for nourishment while exercising when using intermittent fasting:

Early Morning Exercise:
•   Exercise fasted in the early morning: aerobic or anaerobic. Examples: running or weights

•   Take BCAAs afterward - up to 30 grams before lunch.

•   Around Noon: Eat lunch. Aim for about 20-25% of your daily calorie intake.
•   Around 3 PM: Snack on high-fat foods, nuts, and seeds.
•   Between 4-5 PM: Eat dinner. This should be your largest meal of the day.
•   Fast from 8 pm until noon the next day.
Lunch Time Exercise:
•   Just before Noon: Take up to 30 grams of BCAAs.
•   Exercise fasted at lunch: aerobic or anaerobic. Again as examples: running, or weights
•   After exercising around 1-2pm: Eat lunch. Aim for 20-25% of your daily calorie intake.
•   Around 3-4 PM: Snack on high-fat foods, nuts, and seeds
•   Around 6 PM: Eat dinner. This meal's calories should approximate your lunches.

- Around 8-9 PM: Eat something light. Snack if needed.
- Fast from 9 pm or 10 pm until 1-2pm the next day.

You will likely not be working out every single day. So, on rest days, your biggest meal of the day should be your first one instead of your last. On rest days, aim for consuming roughly 35-40% of your calories in your first meal, and eat a lot of protein and fat as part of this meal.

Common Mistakes When Fasting

You still eat unhealthy foods

If you are eating McDonalds every day as a part of your daily meal or meals – depending on which plan you pick – then you have your work cut out for you. You need to switch to unprocessed healthy foods for maximum impact. Try to consume a large meal of wild meat or organic vegetables and see the difference.

This principle extends to beverages too. Stick to water, unsweetened coffee or tea and cut out all the processed juices and carbonated beverages from your diet.

You do not stay busy

Every time someone tells you "hey here is a secret for you to keep" your basic instinct is to go around and tell everyone! Similarly, when you are told, "do not eat food" your unconscious urge is to go and eat everything that you can!

So, when you are fasting, go and find something to do. Go golfing or take a swim. Read a book or watch your favorite show on Netflix (not Master Chef though!) anything to keep you distracted and occupied. Avoid going places where there is bound to be food.
You have too many stimulants

Intermittent Fasting allows you to switch your breakfast for a cup or two of unsweetened coffee. The caffeine keeps you alert, and the coffee fills you up a bit, helping you to feel full for a while. A few cups of coffee before lunch is fine, but don't get addicted to it to the extent that it starts replacing food.

You start out over ambitious

Do not start your Intermittent Fasting journey by directly jumping in with 24-hour fasting; you are just setting yourself up for failure. When you switch from frequently eating to not eating at all (or eating a single meal), it is too severe a change for your body to adjust to. Start out with the 16/8 diet initially, then slowly add in a day of Eat Stop Eat once a week and then shift to a meal a day diet. The slow progression will help your body to adjust to the change, and it will be easier for you.

You are scared of feeling hungry

Feeling hungry is a normal bodily reaction. It doesn't mean that you are starving or your bodily functions will stop, or you will die. Your body is made of a lot of tougher stuff and can easily handle fasting periods of 16 or 20 hours. So do not feel scared, it is just a reaction, and if you ignore it, the pangs will go away.

More is not better

Wow! After fasting for 24 hours I felt so good, why don't I fast for 48 hours? Or even for 72 hours? Well, the benefits of fasting start reducing after a fasting period of 20 hours. There is a thin but firm line that separates fasting from starving, do not cross it!

You are not accepting the chaos

When you make your nutrition consumption schedule a little haphazard, your body goes into a state of chaos and in this state of chaos, whenever you consume anything; the body immediately absorbs all the required nutrients as it is unsure when the next feeding will be. So, Intermittent Fasting provides your body with stress that it needs to learn to cope with slowly and this short-term deprivation just makes your body more efficient. So, when you accept this chaos, you make your body work in a more efficient manner.

You are continuously looking at the clock

You are a human and not a machine. You do not need to do things by the hands of a clock. Eat when you are ready to eat, not when the clock tells you to. If you are very hungry and it is not the time for your meal, munch on a few raw fruits or vegetables. Do not look at the clock but just say it is not dinner time and continue to keep yourself going. Your feeding window is a rough time frame, not an absolute compulsion.

Myths About Intermittent Fasting

Many myths are being shared about intermittent fasting diets and their effectiveness or lack thereof. Looking at some of the more common ones floating around will not only help you in deciding if intermittent fasting is the right weight loss tool for you, but it will prepare you in case you may encounter them in social situations.

1.   Intermittent fasting will slow down your metabolism, making it harder for you to lose weight.
This myth that the frequency of eating your meals will slow down your metabolism and put your body into "starvation mode" is extremely common and well known. There is a ton of research supporting the claim that no matter how many times you're eating per day if the calorie amount is consistent, your rate of metabolism will be unaffected.

2.   Intermittent fasting breaks down muscle in the body to use as energy.
Everyone needs some muscle in their body, even average women who have zero interest in looking like a body builder. Muscle development does impact your metabolic rate, gives you strength, and confidence, and is responsible for the body shape that most women wish to achieve. So, of course, we don't want to do anything that will encourage the body to draw upon muscle mass for energy. Studies have shown that as long as you are using your muscle mass (even in the form of light to moderate physical activity), your muscles will not break down and disappear even in the presence of an extended period of fasting.18

3.   Skipping breakfast makes you gain weight.
Everyone has heard this one! You'll probably hear it a dozen more times while following your intermittent fasting lifestyle. There is a myth that has been around for many years that there is something special about breakfast. So, many men and women falsely believe that skipping breakfast will lead to weight gain. There have been studies done that observed the connection between people who regularly skip breakfast and their weight showing that there is, in fact, a statistical correlation between skipping this meal and being overweight or obese. This is probably explained by the fact that the average person skipping breakfast is less health conscious and nutrition-savvy in general. A study done in 2014 compared overweight and obese subjects who ate breakfast and those who didn't. After 16 weeks, there was no difference in the weight of either group.

4.   Intermittent fasting is bad for your overall health.

Throughout this book, we've looked at numerous evidence-based examples of why this is simply not true. There are a variety of benefits provided to your body from planned and timed fasting including protection against cancer and Alzheimer's disease, weight loss, mental clarity, detoxification of cells within the body, simplification of a diet and nutritional routine, increased energy, and more!

5.   Intermittent fasting will make you overeat, causing you to gain weight.
Some people claim that you won't lose weight using intermittent fasting because you'll overcompensate during your eating periods and eat more than you would normally. This can be true, and some people do tend to eat slightly more after breaking a fast than they would have normally eaten had they not been fasting. An analysis of people following a fasting protocol was studied and showed that those who fasted for an entire 24 hours ended up taking in about 500 extra calories the next day. So, these people expended (or used up) about 2,400 calories during their fasting day, and the next day, they "overcompensated" by consuming an "extra" 500 calories. So, taking all of this information into account, these people had a 1,900 calorie deficit over a 2-day period, which is a substantial deficit in a short period and would lead to significant weight loss. Other studies have shown that fasting for 3–24 weeks (with no dietary changes or exercise included) can decrease belly fat anywhere from 4% to 7% and cause a weight loss of 0.55 lbs–1.65 lbs per week.7

6.   Intermittent fasting is only for men and women who want to be bodybuilders.
This last myth couldn't be farther from the truth! Intermittent fasting is not a diet, and it's not specific to any one gender, type of person, or lifestyle. It's for any person who wants to simplify the complicated world of dieting and nutrition to lose weight and gain overall good health. It doesn't require heavy workouts, intense exercise, or hours of pre-planning meals. It can be easily incorporated into your daily life, whether you work full time or stay at home with your children. There are various methods of intermittent fasting, and the beauty of this weight loss program is that you can use the eating plan that works with your specific schedule and your specific dietary needs!

Do You Want to Live Longer?

I am sure that most people, given a choice, would want to live for a longer time. Many of the unpleasant illnesses that people suffer as they get older are as a result of lifestyle choices. Doctors have even found that illnesses like Alzheimer's can be helped by introducing intermittent fasting. In this chapter, I deal with questions that people ask me about this lifestyle and try to answer them because I am sure you will have questions and I want this book to be completely comprehensive:

How do you know the diet is working?

One of the best things about intermittent fasting is that you feel the benefits pretty soon after starting. For example, when you wake up in the morning, you aren't starving hungry. You learn to accept that the diet is part of your life, but you also have this wonderful feeling of being slimmer even if you don't weigh less. I found that the measurement of my waistline was the first indication that something good was happening. With the diet I used to be on, I used to suffer from a lot of expansion of this area due to the wind and also due to constipation. Giving my body that 16-hour break a day means that it has the chance to repair all of the damage I have done to it over the years.

What do you do when you feel temptation?

I have a good trick for this, which perhaps you can also employ. I try to occupy myself but have a photograph of myself when I was much younger and more attractive. This works as my incentive. If you have found something that inspires you, this helps you to keep motivated. After you have been on this fast over a long period, you know that your cravings are unjustified and can wait that short length of time until midday to sate them. Just find yourself something useful to do instead, and the cravings will slowly disappear into the background.

When is the best time to exercise?

Exercise is always beneficial although I find the best time to exercise is in the morning. I don't do exercise that is too strenuous, but I do enjoy going for a swim or a walk in the morning even if the walk is only to the corner shop. As you become more aware of what you have inflicted on your body over the years, you feel more enthused about exercise because it speeds up the metabolism and it also makes you feel good about your body. If you have been overweight for sometimes, as I was, then you can see that exercise is the way to go because it burns all of that excess fat quicker than diet alone.

Can I eat chocolate?

You can eat most things, but you need to remember your purpose. If your purpose were to lose weight, then you would be healthier choosing dark chocolate without all the milk in it and making one chocolate a real treat instead of a whole packet! Try to think of this as a way of life because that's what you are trying to make it become. You won't deprive yourself of chocolate for always so why even try? Just learn that limitation is the answer to all things. You can have what you like, but in small doses. Remember, it's up to you how much weight you lose and how much exercise you put in. If I find myself eating at the homes of friends and over-indulge, I tend to cut down over the next couple of days or make sure that I put in extra exercise to compensate for it.

Are there any foods that are forbidden?

That depends on how effective you want the diet to be. For example, if you keep on eating fast foods, expect to lose weight slower. Expect your body to object as well because you are introducing a lot of bad stuff to your body and it takes longer to detoxify. I would say that the foods to avoid are:

- Processed foods
- Canned foods with sugar and sodium content
- Foods with too much starch
- An overload of fatty foods

What if I can't drink that much?

People often say that they can't drink that much water, but of course, that's inaccurate. What they are saying is that they don't want to or that they feel uncomfortable drinking that much. When you are on a fast, drinking water is essential. Don't try to drink too much at the same time as this is often where people go wrong. Instead of doing that, allow yourself a sip here and there and have cups of green tea or black coffee occasionally to break the monotony, but do be aware that tea is better than coffee. Coffee takes a lot of the goodness from your body because it acts as a diuretic and while you are on a fast, you do need the goodness of the water you drink to go to the right places in your body. Thus make sure that coffee is only drunk in very small quantities and never use milk or cream during the hours of fasting.

What exercise do you recommend?

Personally, I think it's something you need to examine yourself. Do what gives you pleasure. For example, some people enjoy dancing, and that can give you loads of energy. Others enjoy swimming because it's a low impact exercise that does you so much good and can be done by people of all ages. Walking is also beneficial because it's getting you out and about and if you can walk in a natural environment that's even more beneficial because it tends to lift your spirits and keep you motivated.

Should I prepare to start this diet in advance?

Try and think of it as a lifestyle change. I would say that it is wise to prepare for it. This allows you to buy lots of fresh fruit and vegetables and fresh meats and also to make a note of what you fancy for small snacks. Remember, you can eat more frequently during the eating time and thus will need lots of ideas. Carrot sticks are not the only alternative for snacks. Avoid those snacks that are processed or bought ready to eat. It's much better to make your snacks. Since you need to have the right foods in stock and you will also need to start making a note of your weight and your experiences in journal format, then I would say you need to prepare and then set a date for starting the new lifestyle change. Don't think of it as a diet. The days of diets have finished.

You have chosen to do something to change your lifestyle. If you think of it regarding diet, you will always have the inclination to stop doing it and fasting in this way is something you do for as long as you wish. In fact, I have found most people who take up this style of eating and giving their body the rest that it needs between eating enjoy this lifestyle more than their old lifestyles. Think of it as a change and yes, do prepare for it. If you are doing this with your partner, you need to go through the preparations together, supporting each other in this real change that will help you to lose weight and get rid of toxins that may just be making you old before your time.

Tips to Stay Motivated

Have you managed to shed some weight? And then regain whatever you have managed to shed? Well, it isn't a rocket science to figure it out that you were low on motivation. But then a few weeks into it your motivation starts to falter? Well, don't worry. This is normal. It happens to the best of us. Having the same old boring meals might leave you feeling frustrated and annoyed. You might end up binging on things you have been avoiding for so long. A few slip-ups and you feel emotionally as well as physically derailed. Don't let this get to you. Having the right motivation can help you stick to a diet without having to worry about any distractions. Attitude matters as much as keeping an eye on what you eat and how much you exercise. All your efforts will go for a toss if you don't stay motivated. Going through the process of weight loss will take time, and it does get difficult especially with all the temptations that we are surrounded with.

Set realistic goals

The first thing you need to do while wanting to diet is set goals. You need to be able to maintain your mojo throughout the process and not just during the initial few weeks. One of the factors that have a major impact on whether or not your diet will prove to be a success is the goals you set for yourself. If you are setting goals that are simply unattainable, then you are just setting yourself up for failure. If you set the goal of losing 30 pounds in a month, then that's physically impossible and dangerous as well. Set goals that are attainable. You can set long-term as well as short-term goals. Your short-term goal can be shedding 5 pounds in one month. That's perfectly achievable, and when you achieve the goal you have set for yourself, the chances of you succeeding again are high.

Expect setbacks

You need to understand that it is okay to experience setbacks. A setback isn't a failure it simply means a delay. And every one of us cannot resist temptation every single time. There will be times when you won't be able to resist temptation, and you might give in. The danger isn't about eating something once, but it shouldn't become an excuse for you to binge every single time. Don't think that just because you have gone off track once, you will do it again. Just accept your mistake and ensure that you don't repeat it ever again.

Don't try to be a perfectionist
So, you have managed to gobble down a pint of ice cream or had a cheeseburger for lunch? Don't try to be a perfectionist here. Perfectionist thinking hinders success. If you indulge in a 200-calorie treat, then it is all right and perfectly normal. You are human after all. But this cannot be the reason for giving into a 1000-calorie indulgence just because you

have broken your diet once. If you do slip up, you need to remember that it is perfectly all right. Everyone has their moments once in a while. You need to remember that you should keep going and don't give up.

Buddy system is helpful

It is difficult when you are swimming upstream, especially when you are doing everything all by yourself. It might be really helpful if you have someone else who has got similar goals. Your buddy will provide the support system that you require and will also keep you in check every time you are going off course. It might be really difficult to resist temptation, and when you have someone else by your side who is in the same position as you are, then it will work wonders for yourself confidence. There are various support groups out there that can help you with this.

You will need to be patient

Don't expect any results to happen overnight. The journey of shedding weight will take some time. You will need to be patient. You cannot expect miracles. You will need to follow your diet closely. You will need to exercise regularly and eat right. It will take a while for your efforts to pay off. But they will pay off, and when they do, you will be pleasantly surprised. It is all right even if the results don't show after a week. You will need to stay on track. You can make changes to your diet plan if you think a particular diet isn't working. Just see to it that you aren't going back to your unhealthy ways.

Remember to reward yourself

You need to remember to reward yourself every time you do something right. You can criticize yourself when you do something wrong, but you should also reward yourself whenever you do something right. It needn't be anything expensive. Maybe you can treat yourself to a day out at a spa or probably buy yourself that pair of shoes you have wanted forever. But don't reward yourself with those foods that you aren't supposed to eat. You can set short-term as well as long-term goals and reward yourself whenever you achieve any of your goals.

You will need a maintenance plan

It is an achievement that you have managed to achieve your goal. But your work isn't done, yet. You will need to develop a maintenance plan that will help you ensure that the weight that you have managed to shed keeps off. It is not just about attaining your physical goal, but it is also about maintaining it. You will need to devise a plan that will help you stay on track even in the long run. But it needn't be as strict as your diet plan. For making a plan, you can always consult an expert so that you get the guidance you need.

So, you will need to do everything that you can for staying motivated. Your efforts will pay off. Always remember to keep a positive outlook. Don't let any negativity make you doubt yourself.

Tips and Tricks For A Healthier Lifestyle

If you are planning to start fasting intermittently here are some key pointer to consider.

Don't Try If When at The First Week Of Your Ketogenic/Low-Carb Diet

It's important to note that intermittent fasting should not be tried during the first weeks of ketogenic/low-carb diet or when following a standard American diet. Your body should first adapt to ketogenic diet prior to trying any IF protocol. When you get used to ketogenic diet your body will learn to utilize ketones instead of glucose for energy. Any attempt to start IF straight way will not succeed, instead, your body will become glucose-dependent and this will make you too hungry to follow any IF protocol. Remember intermittent fasting is a gradual process which should be natural not to make you feel hungry or struggle.

Listen To Your Body

When done naturally intermittent fasting delivers fantastic results. Try be as natural as possible when following your IF protocol. For example, when it's time for lunch and you are not hungry, you do not have to eat, skip it. If it's too late to take your dinner, skip it and have a larger breakfast.

However, IF requires a lot of restrictions and control especially during the fasting window. If you are prone to unhealthy eating habits it can be one of the triggers to overindulgence to unhealthy behaviors. Therefore, you should be very careful when trying any of the IF protocols.

Don't Force Yourself

Never deprive or restrict yourself in the name of intermittent fasting, it should be as natural as possible. First train your body to become fat adapted and the hunger sessions will be minimal. The best way of achieving this is starting slow, avoid taking snacks between your meals and as you get used to it tart skipping one of the regular meals, preferably breakfast.

IF is a lifestyle change and to succeed you need to ease your way in. give it a trial run and see if it's something you can comfortably adopt. Try a single plan, for example, try a 24-hour fast or maybe follow partial fasting that will include an eight-hour eating window. If the trial plan works and the experience is tolerable, you can now work with an ongoing plan.

Eat Well When the Feeding Window Opens

Eating well means eating healthy. One of the biggest challenges of intermittent fasting is over-consuming during the feeding window. You do not have to restrict your food intake but it's also healthy to prioritize taking whole foods.

To enjoy the benefits of intermittent fasting you should never counteract the calorie deficit created during the fasting periods. For this reason, you should avoid overzealous bingeing on processed sugars/carbs.

Keep Yourself Busy

A busy schedule will help you to naturally skip meals. Also, avoid spending much of your time near your kitchen because this can tempt you to take a treat even when not feeling hungry. If you immerse yourself in a serious activity your attention will be diverted from cravings and put into good use. This can be of great importance than you ever imagined, just don't let yourself to fall into boredom. Stay engaged and take part in the most energy-intensive tasks.

Understand If Doesn't Fix Everything

IF has the potential to help you live longer and lose weight but you should fully understand that this is just but one of the methods to help your realize your targets. You should consider other factors like sufficient sleep, stress levels, exercise, micronutrients & macronutrients when striving to achieve your targets. IF should never be used as a quick fix for consumption of more than required carbs. It should be done naturally with feeling deprived or restricted.

Create Leverage
The list of the benefits you get from IF is endless. But, you should remember that the magnitude of these benefits during the first few days or weeks will hugely depend on your will power. Human beings are hardwired and the probability of taking an action to avoid pain is 10 times higher than taking action to gain pleasure.

Challenge yourself and play with your mind using 'negative' goals. Just imagine something awful will happen if you fail to fast more often. Creating a leverage will put every part of your body in the mood to fast more naturally.

Every-Other-Day Diet Plan

The alternate days using this plan was established by an assistant professor, Dr. Krista Varady, from the University of Illinois. Women should consume between 500 to 600 calories, and men need to consume more than 400 to 500 calories daily. However, on the feast day, you can eat anything you want and as much as you want.

The plan takes some planning since the diet begins between the hours of noon and 2 pm. These are some of the items to make your day more enjoyable:

The following meal will supply you with roughly 475 calories—depending on the type of soup used.
- ½ cup cooked chicken cooked without the skin and topped/Lemon juice/Fresh-ground pepper
- Bowl of tomato or low-sodium vegetable soup
- 1 ¼ cups of fruit salad

For Men Only: You can have a whole-wheat roll (medium 96-calorie) for a total of 566 calories.

Prepare the salad with pears strawberries, mandarin orange segments, and melon.

Enjoy Lean Beef

Choose a lean piece of beef cut similar to sirloin or tenderloin steak, and enjoy some low-cal side dishes. The basics of the plan are charted for a woman; for a man—add 80 additional calories with a one-cup serving of asparagus with a teaspoon of olive oil for the topping.

For the remainder of the meal, enjoy a three-ounce seared steak with some onions. Top it off with a bit of blue cheese. Serve it with one cup of chard sautéed in 1 teaspoon of olive oil along with a ½ cup of polenta (cornmeal). Use some lemon juice for seasoning.

Substitute with Seafood

You need to consume some omega-3 fatty acids to remain heart-healthy. For men, boost the counts to 553 by enjoying one cup of kale that has been sautéed with olive oil for an additional 102 calories. Flavor the kale with crushed red pepper, red wine vinegar, and garlic.

As a woman (451 calories) enjoy three ounces of sautéed shrimp with jalapenos, garlic, onions, and some tomatoes (fresh and diced) on a bed of ½ cup of brown rice. Place it all in a six-inch corn tortilla. Also, have ¼ of an avocado (chopped) for dessert.

The Choice of No Meat

Women can choose a meatless meal with 473 calories using a whole-wheat pizza crust. As toppings use some black beans, diced tomatoes, barbecue sauce, fresh corn, and shredded mozzarella cheese. Have a bowl of butternut squash soup made using ¾ cup of fruit sorbet and veggie stock.

Men can veg-out with one cup of cauliflower salad for an extra 48 calories using reduced-fat mayonnaise. He could also add ½ cup fruit such as blueberries, ½ cup yogurt if desired. It is best to use the lower fat plain yogurt with the meal.

A Week's Worth of Planning

The logic behind this weekly regimen example involves eating 300 calories on the low-calorie days but can increase to 400 calories if you have an exercise plan in motion. On the brighter side; women can eat 1200 to 1800 calories on the usual days.

The Low-Calorie Count Days

Day 1:

Breakfast

- 1 small slice of deli meat
- 1 six-ounce glass of tomato juice
- ½ cup strawberries

Morning Snack Time

- ¼ cup mixed berries
- 1 tablespoon whey protein
- Blend the ingredients with 3 ice cubes and a cup of water

Lunch

- 1-ounce low-fat cheese
- ½ cup of pickles
- 1-six-ounce cup of tomato juice

Afternoon Snacktime

- 1 tablespoon salad dressing (calorie-free) on one celery stalk

Dinner Time

- Make an omelet using three egg whites, mushrooms, green peppers, and onions.
- For Dessert have ½ cup of strawberries

Evening Snack

- Whey protein smoothie is your savior to enjoy with a cup of mixed veggies.
- Normal Calorie Counted Days

Day 2:

Breakfast

- 1 small banana
- 20 Blueberries
- 1 English muffin (whole wheat) with 2 ¼ teaspoons of peanut butter
- 2/3 cup fat-free yogurt

Morning Snacktime

- 3 saltines
- 1 reduced-fat string cheese stick

Lunch

- 3 tablespoons of hummus with tomato and lettuce
- 1 Whole wheat wrap
- Dessert: 1 cup low-fat yogurt and ½ cup of applesauce

Afternoon Snacktime

- 15 almonds

Dinner

- 3 ounces—chicken breast

- 1 cup of broccoli and 2/3 cup of couscous

Evening Snacks

- 1 tablespoon peanut butter on 2 large graham cracker squares
- Low-Calorie Day
-

Day 3:

Breakfast Meal

- ½ fruit serving
- 1-ounce of protein
- 1 six ounce glass of tomato juice

Mid-morning Snack

- ¼ of a serving of fruit
- Smoothie: Combine three pieces of ice + one cup of water with one tablespoon whey protein.

Lunch Menu

- 1-ounce of protein
- 1 six-ounce glass of tomato juice

Mid-afternoon Snack

- Enjoy something under 50 calories.

Dinner Meal

- No more than 100 calories—include protein, veggies, and fruit as a focus point
- Normal Calorie Count Day
-

Day 4:

Breakfast Meal

- 20 blueberries
- ¼ cup banana
- Whole wheat English muffin with 1 tablespoon of peanut butter

Mid-morning Snack

- 2 tablespoons of light cheese

- 3 rye crackers

Lunch

- 6 whole wheat crackers
- 1 cup of vegetable beef soup
- 1 piece fresh fruit

Mid-Afternoon Snack

- 5-6 medium strawberries
- 1-ounce dark chocolate

Dinner Menu

- Steak and Peppers

Grill or broil:

- 1—four-ounce flank steak flavored with pepper and salt
- Sauté Pepper Mixture:
- 2 teaspoons red wine
- 1 teaspoon olive oil
- ¼ cup onion sliced
- ¾ cup sliced bell pepper
- 1 tablespoon hoisin sauce

Instructions

- Over a medium heat setting, sauté each of the ingredients listed using the teaspoon of olive oil.
- After the flank steak is cooked to your preference, add the sautéed pepper mixture.

Calories: 267 per serving

Safety and Side Effects

Intermittent fasting may not be for everyone. In fact, some people should be careful with intermittent fasting or avoid it altogether. For example, if you are underweight, or have had a history of eating problems and disorders, then you should not do intermittent fasting without first consulting with a health professional. In this type of case, intermittent fasting can do more harm than good.

It has been mentioned, on rare occasions, that it may not be quite as beneficial for women to fast. Albeit rare, it was shown in a rat trial actually to worsen blood sugar control. In addition, there have been a few instances where intermittent fasting can make female rats abnormally thin, weak, masculinized, infertile and cause them to miss cycles. Although no human studies are showing this, it is still important to be aware of this possibility.

Some anecdotal reports from women say they became amenorrheic (their menstrual period stopped) when they first started intermittent fasting, but then it went back to normal once they stopped doing it. Therefore, women should be a little more mindful to their body's reaction when intermittent fasting. My suggestion is that women ease into it, starting with longer eating windows in the range of 10-12 hours and slowly working your way down.

If you are trying to conceive, then consider halting intermittent fasting temporarily. Intermittent fasting is not recommended when pregnant or breastfeeding as it is most important to make sure you have enough proper nutrition to feed yourself and the baby.

While there are numerous benefits to intermittent fasting, I do not recommend this lifestyle for anyone who is underweight or has a history of eating disorders. On the contrary, please seek help from a medical professional to maximize your mental and physical state.

As I stated before, the main side effect of intermittent fasting is hunger. You may feel weak and light headed, but realize that this is only temporary. Once you allow your body time to adapt to using fat as its primary fuel, you will feel better than you did before.

If you have a medical condition, then you should consult with your doctor before trying intermittent fasting. This can include:

- Diabetes
- Blood sugar problems
- Low blood pressure
- Taking medications
- Underweight
- History of eating disorders
- Female and trying to conceive
- Female with a history of amenorrhea
- Pregnant or breastfeeding.

With all that said, intermittent fasting has an outstanding safety profile. If you are a healthy and well-nourished individual, there is nothing dangerous about not eating for a relatively short period.

Conclusions

If you want to stick to intermittent fasting for life, then you must not view it as a diet but as a lifestyle. This will require you to reevaluate your eating choices even before beginning the fast so that when you begin, you are sure that you won't be going back. For example, if you use regular vegetable oil then it is time to replace it with healthy oils such as coconut oil and olive oil. If you tend to eat processed carbs, then it is time to replace them with healthy whole, unprocessed carbs- e.g. zucchini noodles in place of pasta.

The idea here is to embrace the diet and the fact that your body will be a full on fat burning means that new carbs won't be required for body fuel. It will typically take a few weeks for this to happen but once it does, cravings for unhealthy carbs will be out of the picture and incorporating this diet into your life will be as easy as ABC.

If you are going to live the ultimate intermittent fasting lifestyle, then:

The best way to include Intermittent Fasting into your lifestyle is by delaying your breakfast slowly by slowly- delay by an hour then another hour the next day and so on. Take an hour to shower, an hour to do your chores, an hour to get to work- just take an hour from any activity that you engage in the morning that you see best fit until you get to a time that you can live with.

Do not use fasting as an excuse to eat junk- calories are different. 100 calories of broccoli are not the same as 100 calories of a snicker bar. When you find yourself cheating then get real with yourself. Keep the carbs for before workouts and fill yourself up with meats and veggies.

Stick to the method that you are most comfortable with- as discussed; there are a number of ways to do intermittent fasting. Play around with all of them and get what suits you best. Make sure you try out all methods- you might be surprised which will be easiest to follow. To make something part of your lifestyle, you need to be fully comfortable with it. Intermittent fasting is no different.

Intermittent Fasting as a Lifestyle

Guide for you that will help you quickly and easily build up
a Healthy and Beautiful Body

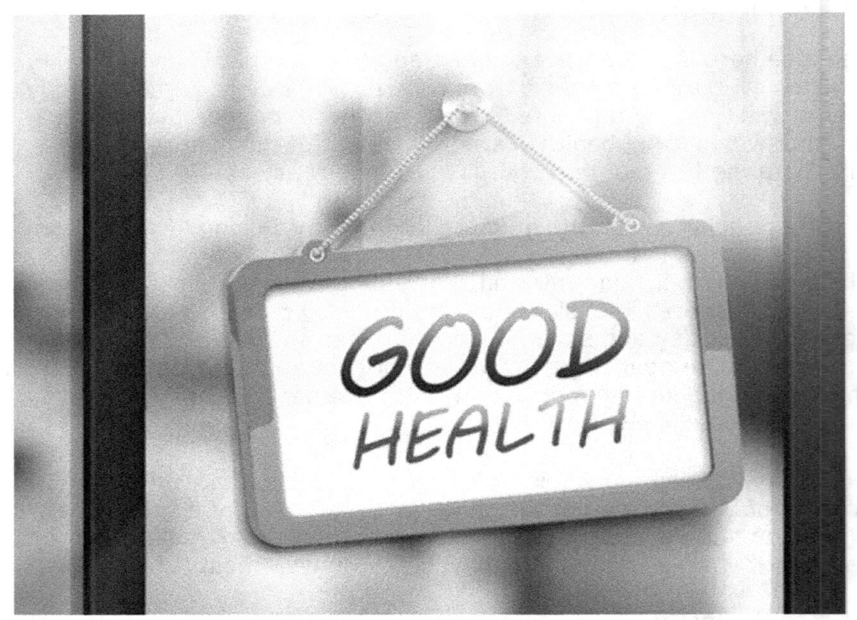

Mia Walker

Your Free Gift

I would like to show my appreciation that you support my work so I've put together a free gift for you that can be found at the link

http://ehpcom.com/.

7 Day-Meal

I know you will love this gift.

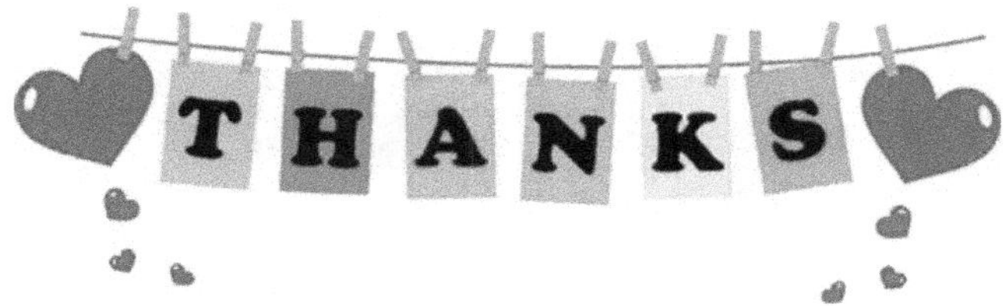

Copyright 2018 by Mia Walker. All rights reserved.